Department of Health

Report on Health and Social Subjects

KU-016-892

49

Nutrition and Bone Health:

with particular reference to calcium and vitamin D

Report of the Subgroup on Bone Health, Working Group on the Nutritional Status of the Population of the Committee on Medical Aspects of Food and Nutrition Policy

London: The Stationery Office

First published 1998

ISBN 0 11 322262 9

Printed in the United Kingdom for The Stationery Office.
J65465, C20, 11/98, 5673.

Preface

The report from the Advisory Group on Osteoporosis was published by the Department of Health in 1994[1]. This expert group asked for further work in specified areas "that guidelines for the treatment of osteoporosis should be prepared, and that further work should be done on preventive measures such as dietary calcium and physical activity". The further work has now been completed and this report from the Committee on Medical Aspects of Food and Nutrition Policy deals particularly with calcium and vitamin D, and to a lesser extent with physical activity, in the public health context. At the same time, the Royal College of Physicians of London has prepared Guidelines for Strategies to Prevent and Treat Osteoporosis, and this report is also being published[2].

In order to consider such a complex question as what factors influence bone health, the Committee on Medical Aspects of Food and Nutrition Policy appointed a new subgroup of experts in this area. I am grateful to Dr Ann Prentice, who chaired the group, and to the members for the work done to prepare this report. Its strength lies in its resolute adherence to scientific integrity and comprehensive assessment of the data both national and international.

I believe that it will provide a sound basis for the development of public health policy.

SIR KENNETH CALMAN
Chairman, Committee on Medical Aspects of Food and Nutrition Policy*

---

* Chairman during preparation of this report, until April 1998

Contents

Committee on Medical Aspects of Food and Nutrition Policy

Working Group on the Nutritional Status of the Population: Subgroup on the Nutritional Aspects of Bone Health

Chairman

Dr Ann Prentice   MRC Dunn Nutrition Unit, Cambridge

Members

Professor P J Aggett	Lancashire Postgraduate School of Medicine and Health, University of Central Lancashire; formerly Institute of Food Research and Norwich and Norfolk Hospital
Dr C Bolton-Smith	Ninewells Hospital and Medical School, University of Dundee
Professor M Chan	Department of Public Health, Liverpool (formerly Director, NHS Ethnic Health Unit, Leeds
Professor C Cooper	MRC Environmental Epidemiology Unit, Southampton
Professor Sir John Grimley Evans	Division of Geriatric Medicine, Nuffield Department of Clinical Medicine, University of Oxford
Professor A Shenkin	Department of Clinical Chemistry, University of Liverpool

Observers

Professor M J Wiseman	Department of Health, London
Dr R Harding (until Sept 1996)	Ministry of Agriculture, Fisheries and Food, London

Dr D Kennedy (from Oct 1996)   Ministry of Agriculture, Fisheries and Food, London

Secretariat

Dr P C Clarke (Medical)   Department of Health, London

Ms D Alexander (Scientific)
(until April 1997)   Department of Health, London

Ms H Lee (Scientific)
(from June 1997)   Department of Health, London

Committee on Medical Aspects of Food and Nutrition Policy

Working Group on the Nutritional Status of the Population

Chairman

Professor P J Aggett   Lancashire Postgraduate School of Medicine and Health, University of Central Lancashire; formerly Institute of Food Research and Norwich and Norfolk Hospital

Members

Dr D H Buss*   Nutrition Consultant, Hampshire

Professor Sir John Grimley Evans   Division of Geriatric Medicine, Nuffield Department of Clinical Medicine, University of Oxford

Professor A A Jackson   Department of Human Nutrition, University of Southampton

Dr Ann Prentice   MRC Dunn Nutrition Unit, Cambridge

Professor A Shenkin   Department of Clinical Chemistry, University of Liverpool

Observers

Professor M J Wiseman   Department of Health, London

Dr R Harding (until Sept 1996)   Ministry of Agriculture, Fisheries and Food, London

Miss E J Wordley
(Oct 1996-June 1997)   Ministry of Agriculture, Fisheries and Food, London

Mr W Scriven
(from July 1997)   Ministry of Agriculture, Fisheries and Food, London

---

* d. 29 August 1998

Committee on Medical Aspects of Food and Nutrition Policy

Chairman

Sir Kenneth Calman
(until April 1998)

Chief Medical Officer, Department of Health

Members

Professor P J Aggett

Lancashire Postgraduate School of Medicine and Health, University of Central Lancashire; formerly Institute of Food Research and Norwich and Norfolk Hospital

Dr S Bingham

MRC Dunn Clinical Nutrition Centre, Cambridge

Professor G Fowler

Professor Emeritus of General Practice, University of Oxford

Professor Sir John Grimley Evans

Division of Geriatric Medicine, Nuffield Department of Clinical Medicine, University of Oxford

Professor A A Jackson

Department of Human Nutrition, University of Southampton

Professor W P T James

Director, Rowett Research Institute, Aberdeen

Professor M G Marmot

Department of Epidemiology and Public Health, University College, London

Professor D P Richardson

Nestlé UK Limited, Croydon

Dr P Troop

Anglia and Oxford Regional Office

Dr A F Williams

St George's Hospital, London

Assessors

Dr H Campbell	Chief Medical Officer, DHSS Northern Ireland
Professor Sir David Carter	Chief Medical Officer, Department of Health, Scottish Office
Dr Ruth Hall	Chief Medical Officer, Welsh Office
Dr A Peatfield	Medical Research Council
Mr G Podger	Ministry of Agriculture, Fisheries and Food
Ms L Stockley	Health Education Authority

Acknowledgements

The Subgroup is grateful for the written contributions submitted by the following organisations and individuals.

Dr M Alfaham*	Llandough Hospital
Dr E J Bassey* †	Department of Physiology and Pharmacy, University of Nottingham
Dr I Bell	Kelloggs, Manchester
Dr V Burley*	Leeds
Dr J Buttriss	National Dairy Council, London
Ms J Collins*	Nutrition Unit, Ministry of Agriculture, Fisheries and Food, London
Ms T Dean*	Department of Nutrition and Dietetics, King's College, London
Professor R Eastell*	Department of Human Metabolism and Clinical Biochemistry, University of Surrey
Ms N Evans	Chessington, Surrey
Dr R M Francis*	Musculo-Skeletal Department, Freeman Hospital
Dr R Fraser*	Centre for Pregnancy Nutrition, University of Sheffield
Dr W D Fraser*	Department of Clinical Chemistry, University of Liverpool
Ms J Higgs	Meat and Livestock Commission, Milton Keynes
Mr T Lobstein	The Food Commission (UK) Ltd.
Professor B Mawer*	Department of Medicine, University of Manchester

Mr J Murray	The Incorporated National Association of British and Irish Millers Ltd.
Dr S A New	School of Biological Sciences, University of Surrey, Guildford
Dr J Reeve*	MRC Bone Disease Research Group, University of Cambridge
Ms R Rowe	National Osteoporosis Society, Bath
Ms J Scott	Food and Drink Federation, London
Mr P R Sherratt	Salt Manufacturers' Association, Manchester
Mrs M Wynn	London

---

* Submission of expert evidence was requested by COMA.
† Presented oral evidence.

Definition of terms

Body Mass Index (BMI):	An indirect measure of body fatness = weight $(kg)/height (m)^2$.
Bone density:	the density of bone in a skeletal unit (g/cm^3), including bone matrix, mineral, soft tissues (often confused with bone mineral density).
Bone mass:	the mass of bone in a skeletal unit (g), including bone matrix, mineral, soft tissues.
Bone mineral content (BMC):	the mass of bone mineral in a skeletal unit (g).
Bone mineral density (BMD):	the density of bone mineral in a skeletal unit (g/cm^3); when measured by absorptiometry it represents the mass of bone mineral in a scanned area (g/cm^2) and is not a true density measurement.
Bone modelling:	the processes of bone formation and growth.
Bone remodelling:	the structured sequence of events by which old bone is replaced by new bone which involves resorption followed by formation and mineralisation.
Bone remodelling transient:	an incremental change in measured bone mineral content/density caused by an alteration in bone remodelling rate.
Bone turnover:	the replacement of old bone by new bone.
Calciotropic hormone:	a hormone involved in the regulation of calcium homeostasis.
Calcitonin:	hormone secreted by the C-cells of the thyroid, involved in the regulation of calcium homeostasis and other functions.
Calcidiol:	25-hydroxyvitamin D produced in the liver.
Calcitriol:	$1,25(OH)_2$ vitamin D; hormone secreted by the kidney involved in the regulation of calcium homeostasis and other functions.
Calcium binding proteins:	proteins involved in the intestinal absorption of calcium.
Cartilage:	stiff, load bearing tissue: during early life, a cartilage model of a bone precedes its transformation into mature bone tissue, a process which is only completed at maturity when growth ceases.
Chondrogenesis:	cartilage formation.
Collagen:	the principal protein of the bone matrix.

Cortical/compact bone:	dense compact bone with a low surface area: mass ratio providing strength and structure to the skeleton.
Epiphysis:	place where bone begins to be laid down, especially at each end of a long bone; during growth it is separated from shaft of long bone (diaphysis) by cartilagenous plate.
Incidence:	the number of new cases of a disease occurring in a given size of population during a specific period of time, usually a year.
Intervention studies:	an investigation involving intentional change in some aspect of the status of the subjects. The intervention can be at the individual or community/population level.
Odds ratio:	the ratio of odds of exposure to non-exposure among the diseased (cases) compared to the non-diseased (controls) in case-control studies. The odds ratios derived in case-control studies are approximately equivalent to the relative risks (qv) determined in cohort studies.
Osteoblast:	bone forming cell.
Osteocalcin:	non-collagenous bone protein measured in plasma as an index of bone formation rate.
Osteoclast:	bone resorbing cell.
Osteocyte:	cell in the connective tissue of bone.
Osteoid:	uncalcified bone tissue, bone matrix.
Osteomalacia:	skeletal disease characterised by inadequate or delayed mineralisation of bone matrix (osteoid).
Osteon:	concentric cylinders of collagen fibres and mineral crystals in bone tissue.
Osteonectin:	a non-collagenous bone protein.
Osteoporosis:	skeletal disease characterised by low bone mass and micro-architectural deterioration.
Parathyroid hormone (PTH):	hormone secreted by the parathyroid glands involved in the regulation of calcium homeostasis and other functions.
Peak bone mass:	the maximum bone mass achieved by mid-life.
Prevalence:	the number of cases observed in a given size of population at a designated time.
Pseudofractures/Looser's zones:	focal accumulation of osteoid, a diagnostic feature of osteomalacia.
Rickets:	disease of the immature skeleton characterised by inadequate mineralisation of bone matrix (osteoid).
Trabecular/cancellous bone:	spongy bone with a high surface area: mass ratio found principally at the end of the long bones, and within the axial skeleton.

Abbreviations

mole:	molecular weight in grams
nmol:	nanomole or 10^{-9} mole or one-thousand-millionth of mole
g:	gram
mg:	milligram or 10^{-3} g or one-thousandth of 1g
µg:	microgram or 10^{-6} g or one-millionth of 1g
pg:	picogram or 10^{-12} g or one-million-millionth of 1g
l:	litre
IU:	International Units. Used to quantify vitamin D dose. For defining dosage of vitamin D both International Units and metric weights are used. 1 International Unit (IU) = 0.025 µg crystalline vitamin D_3 i.e. 1 µg = 40 IU vitamin D_3
y:	year
d:	day
25(OH)vitamin D:	25-hydroxyvitamin D (occurs almost exclusively in plasma); calcidiol nmol/l (0.4006) = µg/l
1,25(OH)$_2$vitamin D:	1,25 dihydroxyvitamin D (the active form of the vitamin involved in calcium homeostasis); calcitriol pmol/l (0.4167) = ng/l
PTH:	parathyroid hormone nmol/l (2.516) = µg/l
DRV:	Dietary Reference Value
EAR:	Estimated Average Requirement
RNI:	Reference Nutrient Intake
LRNI:	Lower Reference Nutrient Intake
MAFF:	Ministry of Agriculture, Fisheries and Food
COMA:	Committee on Medical Aspects of Food and Nutrition Policy
BMD:	bone mineral density
BMC:	bone mineral content

1. Recommendations of the report

Recommendations (Chapter 11)

1.   A healthy lifestyle to maintain bone health should be encouraged at all ages. A varied and adequate diet and regular weight bearing physical activity appropriate for the individual are beneficial. An adequate vitamin D status can be achieved from exposure of the skin to summer sunlight although this needs to be balanced against increasing the risk of skin cancer. Local public health policies should integrate these recommendations in their plans for improving the health of their population[3,4].

2.   No change is recommended in the existing UK Dietary Reference Values for calcium because of insufficient evidence. Recent data do not support the increment for lactation which might not be necessary.

3.   Dietary means of achieving an adequate calcium intake, as assessed against Dietary Reference Values, should be encouraged.

4.   The present policy of fortifying flour with calcium should continue.

5.   The existing UK Dietary Reference Values for vitamin D are endorsed.

6.   The public and health professionals should be better informed about the importance of achieving adequate vitamin D status, including the appropriate use of vitamin supplements for those most at risk of vitamin D deficiency. The most vulnerable groups include:

- infants, young children and pregnant women from Asian families as well as young African-Caribbean children being reared on strict exclusion diets;

- older people who are housebound, who live in institutions or who eat no meat or oily fish;

- and people who rarely go out of doors or who, when they do so, wear clothes which fully conceal them.

7.   Local health authorities and health professionals should be aware that sporadic cases of clinical vitamin D deficiency still occur. They should be alert to the possibilities of inadequacies in their population from knowledge of the social and cultural antecedents of vitamin D deficiency and should consider instituting appropriate community-based preventive programmes.

8.   The statutory requirement to fortify margarine with vitamin D should be maintained; reduced fat spreads should also be fortified with vitamin D but providing the majority of manufacturers continue to do this on a voluntary basis there is no need for this to be a statutory requirement.

9.   Maintenance of a healthy body weight at all ages should be encouraged. Being underweight is particularly detrimental to bone health.

10.   A lifestyle which includes regular physical activity, particularly that which is weight bearing, should be encouraged at all ages, and a sedentary lifestyle discouraged.

Recommendations for research

11.   More research is needed into the influence on bone of individual nutrients including calcium and vitamin D as well as other nutrients.

12.   The mechanisms underlying nutritional effects on bone should be clarified. This should include studies on the effects of endocrine and growth factors and their interaction in the balance between bone synthesis and bone resorption at the different stages of life in women and men.

13.   Interactions between diet, body composition, physical activity, and bone status require more study.

14.   The long term relationship between measures of bone status during childhood and adolescence, and peak bone mass in adulthood and bone health in old age should be clarified.

15.   Well controlled intervention studies with long term follow-up of the clinical effects on bone should be set up to investigate the influence of diet and lifestyle on bone health in well characterised populations throughout the age range.

16.   In respect to calcium and vitamin D, the mechanisms and limitations of the adaptive response to different diets with particular emphasis on inter-individual variations, nutrient-gene interactions and the importance of the environment in early life should be investigated further.

17.   The effect of seasonal variations in vitamin D status on osteoporosis should be investigated, and the mechanisms involved identified.

18.   The public health aspects of exposure to sunlight should be defined urgently to take account of the importance of this source of vitamin D relative to increasing the risk of skin cancer.

19.   For those needing vitamin D supplementation, the most acceptable, efficient and cost effective way of providing it, should be identified.

20.   Nationally representative data on nutritional status and dietary intakes in Britain should continue to be collected to monitor trends where inadequacies such as low vitamin D status have previously been found and to identify vulnerable groups.

21.   There should be continued surveillance of minority groups at risk of vitamin D inadequacy or of low dietary calcium intakes. The characteristics of those groups should be more fully identified.

22.   The present programme of diet and nutrition surveys should be extended to include pregnant women and infants and also to collect more detailed information about physical activity levels where possible.

23.   Better markers of nutritional status in respect of bone health should be developed for population surveillance.

2. Introduction

2.1 Background

2.1.1   There has long been concern about increasing rates of fractures in the UK, particularly hip, wrist and vertebral fractures, which have been attributed to osteoporosis[5]. Over 200,000 fractures a year, the majority in older people, cost the National Health Service over £940 million. Fractures are more common in women, and more common in white populations than in populations of African or Caribbean origins. It is estimated that around 60,000 hip fractures and 50,000 wrist fractures occur annually in the United Kingdom[2]. About 40,000 vertebral fractures are diagnosed clinically per year, but this represents only a proportion of the total with possibly as many as two thirds not coming to medical attention[1]. The social and personal burdens of pain and disability attributable to osteoporosis are substantial.

2.1.2   There are higher fracture rates in Europe and North America when compared with other countries, and in Europe there is a declining gradient from north to south. Fracture rates increase with age, and as the number of old people in the population has increased so has the number of fractures presenting for treatment. This increase was very marked during the 1970s but reached a plateau during the 1980s[6,7]. There was also an increase in age specific fracture rates which suggests that environmental factors may have contributed to the risk in age cohorts. This observation has fuelled several etiological hypotheses which focus on decreasing physical activity (para 7.6), increasing adult height[6], changes in smoking habits (para 7.5), and others. There has been a search for dietary factors which might be implicated, especially milk consumption (para 5.4.6), but no consistent patterns have been defined. The relationship between high latitude and high risk of fracture in Europe suggests that vitamin D insufficiency may be an adverse factor in the development of osteoporosis and this is beginning to be explored (para 6.4.10).

2.1.3   It has been recognised for over 70 years that there are two ways of ensuring an adequate vitamin D status in humans, from the effect of sunlight on the skin in synthesising this vitamin, and by dietary means. In the early parts of the century, poor people living in tenements, overhung by a smoke-laden atmosphere were deprived of sunlight. Nevertheless, the eradication of vitamin D deficiency became a realistic public health goal when Chick and co-workers demonstrated in 1923 that cod liver oil cured rickets[8]. Rickets, which affects infants and children whose bones are growing, and osteomalacia, which affects adults whose bone growth is completed, while now rare in this country, continue to be reported sporadically (Dr R J Harris - personal communication[9,10]). There are usually special factors which contribute to increasing the risk, for example, toddlers being brought up in households which follow very strict Rastafarian practices[9], and infants born to mothers who customarily wear very concealing clothes[10]. A report from COMA in 1980 on rickets and osteomalacia particularly addressed the vitamin D status of people living in the UK who had come from the Indian subcontinent[11]. This recognised the particular cultural and social characteristics which increase the risk of vitamin D deficiency: a diet which excludes meat and fish, a lifestyle of rarely going out of doors, and then wearing concealing clothing, times of increased metabolic demand for vitamin D such as pregnancy and in the early years of life. A campaign of prevention through education and dietary supplementation of target groups, called Stop Rickets, followed the COMA report and was in large measure successful in leading to a decline in the numbers of cases of overt clinical deficiency[12].

2.1.4   Newer biochemical techniques have now allowed improved assessment of vitamin D status and, using these measures, pockets of vitamin D deficiency continue to be reported. A high proportion of Asians, such as has been reported from Leicester, continue to have a poorer vitamin D status, as a group, when compared with the rest of the population[13], and also pregnant Asian women in South Wales[14]. These findings suggest that a proportion of the population of this country is insufficient in vitamin D, although not manifesting the syndromes of clinical deficiency and that the current public health programmes for identifying and advising those at high risk have not been fully effective.

2.1.5   *Department of Health Advisory Group on Osteoporosis*   In 1994, an expert Advisory Group on Osteoporosis[1] recommended that:

"The Committee on Medical Aspects of Food Policy (COMA) should be asked to consider the role of diet in the prevention of osteoporosis, with particular reference to Dietary Reference Values for calcium and vitamin D. Developing knowledge on the value of vitamin D with or without calcium supplementation in the elderly, particularly those living in institutions, means that new advice is needed which should then be implemented at the earliest opportunity".

This new report from COMA responds to the recommendation from the Advisory Group on Osteoporosis. A second recommendation was that the Royal College of Physicians should work with an intercollegiate group to prepare nationally agreed multi-disciplinary clinical guidelines on the prevention and treatment strategies to be incorporated into the Department of Health's clinical effectiveness programme. These guidelines will be published in 1998[2].

2.1.6   *Recommendations on Optimal Bone Health from a USA National Institutes of Health Consensus Panel*   The USA National Institutes of Health (NIH) also published a report in 1994 from a Consensus Development Panel on Optimal Calcium Intake[15]. This made recommendations for higher population calcium intakes than had been indicated by either the USA Recommended Dietary Allowance[16] or the UK Dietary Reference Values[17]. COMA's review of the latest data about the influence of calcium and vitamin D on bone status is therefore timely.

2.1.7   *Statutory fortification of foods*   Margarine has been fortified with vitamin D since the 1920s. During the second world war fortification became required by law which for the past 50 years has been at a level of 7.05-8.82 µg vitamin D per 100g and with vitamin A at a level of 800-1000 µg retinol per 100g and is currently regulated by the Spreadable Fats (Marketing Standards) Regulations 1995 (SI 1995, No 3116). Previous reports from COMA in 1980 (para 2.1.3)[11] and in 1991[18] had been asked to review the need for mandatory fortification of yellow fats and on both occasions recommended that it should continue. In 1994, the Ministry of Agriculture, Fisheries and Food (MAFF) asked the Department of Health for advice on the public health implications of removing the current regulations on compulsory fortification of flour and of margarine. Statutory fortification was an issue considered in the context of the Food Law Deregulation Plan in 1993. Concerns both for and against the continuation of statutory fortification were raised and it was decided that the existing requirements for the fortification of bread and flour, and margarine should be maintained whilst the nutritional significance of the current arrangements for fortification was examined by COMA.

2.1.8   With the outbreak of the Second World War, there were concerns that the national diet might not provide sufficient calcium. It was anticipated that milk and dairy products would become scarce. At the same time in order to conserve such wheat as was available, the extraction rate of flour for bread making was raised to 85 per cent, and subsequently to 90 per cent in 1946. It was argued that this would leave a higher residue in the flour of phytates and other molecules which would bind the calcium in unabsorbable complexes. Since 1943, all wheat flour, except wholemeal, has been required to have calcium carbonate added at the rate of 235-390mg calcium carbonate per 100g flour (equivalent to 94-156mg calcium per 100g flour). Fortification of flour, except wholemeal and certain other specified types, with iron, calcium, thiamin and niacin is mandatory under the Bread and Flour Regulations 1998 (SI 1998, No 141). Further expert reports to Government[19,20] have recommended that compulsory fortification of flour was no longer necessary but it remains in force.

2.2   Committee on Medical Aspects of Food and Nutrition Policy
In response COMA set up the following expert groups.

2.2.1   *Working Group on the Nutritional Status of the Population* was set up in 1995 with the following terms of reference:

"To review the dietary intakes and nutritional status of the population with regard to folic acid and the nutrients currently statutorily added to flour and yellow fats;

• to consider mechanisms, including fortification of foods, for the maintenance of adequate nutritional status and evaluation of their safety and effectiveness;

• to make recommendations on the above;

- to advise on a programme of work to review the dietary intakes and nutritional status of the population with regard to other nutrients."

2.2.2   *Subgroup on Nutrition and Bone Health*   This was set up in 1996 with the following terms of reference:

"To review the dietary intakes and nutritional status of the population with regard to bone health with particular reference to calcium and vitamin D and to make recommendations."

2.2.3   *Meetings of the Subgroup and way of working*   The first of 5 meetings was held on 1 February 1996. The draft report was reviewed by the Subgroup and its parent committee the Working Group on the Nutritional Status of the Population at a joint meeting on 7 July 1997. The final text was approved at the meeting of COMA in April 1998 and thereafter by correspondence.

2.2.4   The Press Release, which announced the setting up of these expert groups, invited submissions of evidence; those received are acknowledged earlier. Dr Victoria Burley was commissioned to review the published data about diet and nutrient intakes for calcium and vitamin D. Ms Tracy Dean of King's College, London, collated recent information about vitamin D deficiency in children aged under 10 years. She reported personal contributions from health professionals in areas where cases of clinical rickets and osteomalacia are still seen in Leicester[21], Bristol[9] and London[22,23], (Dr R J Harris, Royal London Hospital Trust*, Professor J O'Readon, University College Hospital Trust*, Dr V F Larcher, Queen Elizabeth Hospital for Children*) and areas where rickets was no longer seen although vitamin D deficiency had once been widespread in the local Asian community in Glasgow[24], and West Midlands[25].

---

* personal communication

3.   Bone and bone health

3.1   The function of bone

3.1.1   Bone supports and protects the tissues of the body and it provides a framework to enable body movements. It also has metabolic functions which are crucial for the maintenance of life including the homeostasis of ionised calcium in the blood. Within cells calcium ions are essential for the maintenance of the internal cellular structure and the passage of impulses and signals within and between cells. Calcium ions also contribute to a wide range of metabolic functions as well as other complex interactions such as blood clotting. The extracellular fluid concentrations of ionised calcium are strictly maintained and this metabolic call on the calcium in bone has priority.

3.2   The structure of bone

3.2.1   Bone is a highly vascular connective tissue enclosed by a fibrocellular layer, the periosteum. In common with other connective tissues, it consists of a matrix with embedded cells, known as osteocytes, which are scattered but interconnected by extensions to form a cellular network. The matrix consists of collagen fibres usually arranged in parallel and a mineralised ground substance. Bone collagen is strongly cross-linked internally which provides gaps between its fibres. Bone crystals resemble hydroxyapatite $(Ca_{10} (PO_4)_6 (OH)_2)$. In addition to Ca^{++}, PO_4^{---}, and OH^- ions, bone mineral contains numerous other ions such as HPO_4^{--}, CO_3^{--}, F^-, Mg^{++}, Na^+ and citrate that are incorporated in the crystal lattice or adsorbed on the surface. Bone crystals are packed between the collagen fibres to create the characteristic mineralised tissue. Within the bone tissue most of the collagen fibres and the mineral crystals are arranged around neurovascular channels in concentric cylinders known as osteons. The central canal which carries the capillaries within the osteon has numerous perforations which provide pathways for the diffusion of fluids, nutrients and gases.

3.2.2   Both osteoblasts and osteoclasts originate in the bone marrow; the osteoblast derives from mesenchymal stem cells and the osteoclast from the mononuclear/phagocytic cell lineage. The production of these bone cells is partly governed by cytokines which are themselves modulated by sex hormones. The osteoblast is the primary bone forming cell. It is protein synthesising and secretes collagen and a wide range of non-collagenous proteins which, with other organic components, create osteoid, which is uncalcified pre-bone tissue. Osteoblasts facilitate the calcification of the osteoid through a mechanism not yet fully elucidated but involving the secretion, among other factors, of bone-specific alkaline phosphatase, osteocalcin and osteonectin. The precipitation of hydroxyapatite crystals from the matrix fluids is also dependent on a number of other factors including inorganic ion concentrations and local pH. Some osteoblasts become embedded in the matrix of bony tissue to become osteocytes. Osteoclasts are phagocytic cells responsible for removing bone tissue. These cells are rich in lysosomes and they are able to resorb collagen and then absorb matrix debris by pinocytosis. The balanced activity of osteoblasts and osteoclasts provide the means for rapid release and resorption of calcium ions, the repair of injuries to the bone tissue and alterations in bone architecture in response to mechanical stress.

3.2.3   About 80 per cent of the skeleton comprises cortical (compact) bone and 20 per cent trabecular (cancellous) bone. There is heterogeneity between bones, thus, for instance, there is less trabecular bone in the shaft of humerus and more in a vertebral body. Although constituted from the same cells and matrix, cortical and trabecular bone differ in structure and in function. The strength of cortical bone arises because 80-90 per cent of its volume is mineralised. Strength in trabecular bone is provided by internal bracing with struts and girders of bony tissue (the trabeculae). This arrangement gives the advantage of strength with relatively light weight. Bone marrow fills the spaces between the trabeculae of all bones. Red bone marrow is a highly vascular haemopoietic tissue which, by adulthood, is limited to the vertebrae, sternum, ribs, clavicles, scapulae, pelvis, cranial bones and the proximal femora and humeri. Other bones are filled with yellow marrow composed mostly of fat cells.

3.3   **The metabolism of bone**

3.3.1   Bone is a dynamic tissue which is regulated by hormones, growth factors and other chemical mediators. Genetic influences on bone are also beginning to be explored (para 7.1). In childhood, the skeleton is modelled to meet the needs for growth and strength. Growth in length of bones occurs in the layer of epiphyseal cartilage (the growth plate) by a process of chondrogenesis followed by ossification. This ceases at maturity. Growth in width of bones occurs by intramembranous or sub-periosteal bone formation and continues at a slow rate throughout life while endosteal resorption also continues over the lifespan so that, although bones get wider, their cortex gets thinner. These processes constitute modelling. With maturity, changes to the skeleton are achieved through remodelling which is a continuous process of replacement and repair called "bone turnover". It operates to renew ageing bone, to remove fatigue fractures, to adapt the skeleton to physical stress related to physical activity and load bearing, and to release ionised calcium as needed.

3.3.2   *Bone remodelling*   Bone remodelling on the external and internal surfaces of bone is a lifelong process. It occurs throughout the skeleton but is particularly dominant in trabecular bone which has ten times the surface area of compact bone. Initially osteoclasts excavate a resorption pit. Thereafter osteoblasts are attracted and migrate to line the pit. These cells create an osteoid matrix which fills the pit and which is subsequently mineralised. In young adults, the creation of resorption pits with release of calcium is matched by the calcification of newly formed osteoid repairs to earlier pits. There is thus no substantial net change in calcium balance[26]. In particular circumstances, such as

9

the menopause, an increase in the rate of bone resorption leads to the creation of many more resorption pits but bone formation fails to increase sufficiently to restore the lost bony tissue completely. This results in an overall loss of bone (osteoid, cells and mineral) from the skeleton and this is more rapid in trabecular bone because of its greater surface area[27]. A similar situation arises without an increase in bone resorption if bone formation is impaired and with loss of stress/weight bearing activity. When bone loss is severe, as in osteoporosis, the slender trabeculae can be breached resulting in a disconnected structure and loss of strength.

3.3.3   *Bone remodelling transient*   Calcium concentrations in the body's extracellular fluids affect the skeleton. A fall in ionised calcium leads to secretion of parathyroid hormone (PTH) and an increase in the number of resorption pits being excavated at any one time. This results in loss of bone with release of calcium, along with matrix components, which assists in the maintenance of normal extracellular ionised calcium concentrations. Conversely, an increase in ionised calcium results in a decrease in the number of resorption pits excavated and, since new osteoid in previously excavated pits will continue to be laid down and to mineralise, calcium is removed from the circulation and helps to normalise ionised calcium in the extracellular fluids. In the balance state, these changes in bone resorption are matched by equivalent changes in bone formation and, after a period of time, the pits are refilled and the bone completely restored. As there is a time interval between the excavation of each pit and its complete restoration (which can be as much as 4-8 months in cortical bone), a decrease in bone resorption rate will result in a temporary net increase in bone mass until the steady state is re-established. Similarly an increase in bone resorption rate will produce a net decrease. This phenomenon is referred to as the bone remodelling transient[28,29,26]. Calcium supplements have been used in older people with established osteoporosis in an attempt to slow the progress of the disease. However, the clinical significance at any age of a short term increase in bone mineral content as a result of alterations in bone remodelling rate is unknown. Few studies have examined the mechanism underlying the response to changes in calcium intake or have investigated long term benefit, but several are in progress.

3.3.4   *Metabolic effects of changes in calcium and vitamin D status*   Calcium-ion-sensing receptors on membranes of cells in the parathyroid gland, thyroid gland and kidney tubules are responsive to changes in the level of ionised calcium in the extracellular fluid[30]. When ionised calcium concentration falls, PTH output increases which liberates calcium from bone by increasing the number of resorption pits. PTH also stimulates the renal synthesis of $1,25(OH)_2$vitamin D. At customary dietary intakes, intestinal absorption of calcium is by active transport, which is vitamin D dependent, as well as by passive diffusion. $1,25(OH)_2$vitamin D enhances the active phase of absorption by stimulating the synthesis of calcium binding proteins. At the same time renal calcium reabsorption increases. If the level of ionised calcium is raised, PTH secretion is inhibited, calcitonin may be secreted by the thyroid gland and plasma calcium falls. The mechanism underlying these effects is incompletely understood.

3.3.5   Plasma concentration of $1,25(OH)_2$vitamin D is regulated too closely to be a sensitive measure of vitamin D status. The most commonly used index of status is plasma 25(OH)vitamin D which reflects both skin synthesis and dietary intake. At all ages, from neonates[31] to older people[32], lower plasma levels of 25(OH)vitamin D are associated with higher levels of PTH. Low plasma phosphate and raised chloride levels characterise the early stages of vitamin D inadequacy. If compensation fails, the level of alkaline phosphatase usually rises and eventually calcium may fall. Although very low levels of plasma 25(OH)vitamin D are associated with clinical disease (see para 3.4.2), there is less certainty over the clinical implications of levels which, while still low, fall short of those seen in overt metabolic bone disorders which may or may not be associated with higher plasma PTH, or with adverse effects on bone health (see 6.2). There is evidence that low calcium intakes may increase the requirement for vitamin D, since increased breakdown of 25(OH)vitamin D has been demonstrated in calcium-deficient rats[33] and children with calcium-responsive rickets have been documented in South Africa and elsewhere[34].

3.3.6   The secretion of PTH exhibits a circadian rhythm in healthy men and premenopausal women[35,36] with higher levels at night. There is strong correlation between the circadian rhythms for PTH and serum phosphate[37] which are attenuated in established postmenopausal osteoporosis. This loss of a diurnal fall in PTH may contribute to bone loss in these patients[38]. In osteoporotic patients daily injections of PTH at physiological levels have an anabolic effect on human bone[39]. This suggests that the nocturnal rise in PTH as part of the circadian rhythm may have an anabolic effect. Since this rhythm can be modified by varying the dietary intakes of calcium, phosphate and carbohydrate[40], it is possible that the times of day at which these nutrients are eaten may be important in the aetiology or treatment of osteoporosis.

3.4   Clinical presentations: osteoporosis and vitamin D deficiency

3.4.1   Osteoporosis

3.4.1.1 *Osteoporosis*   Osteoporosis is a progressive systemic skeletal disorder characterised by low bone mass and micro-architectural deterioration of bone tissue with a consequent increase in bone fragility and risk of fracture. There is proportionate loss of all bone elements, cells, osteoid and mineral. The definition proposed by a World Health Organization expert group in 1994[41] was:

"A disease characterised by low bone mass and micro-architectural deterioration of bone tissue, leading to enhanced bone fragility and a consequent increase in fracture risk".

The categories of the disease are defined in terms of bone mineral mass or density as follows:

Normal - a value for bone mineral content (BMC) or bone mineral density (BMD) within one standard deviation (sd) of the young adult reference mean for that gender. (There are no absolute standard values other than locally derived population means.)

Low Bone Mass (osteopenia) - a value for BMC or BMD more than one sd below the young adult mean but less than 2.5 sd below this value.

Osteoporosis - a value for BMC or BMD 2.5 sd or more below the young adult mean.

3.4.2 Clinical presentations of vitamin D deficiency

3.4.2.1 *Osteomalacia*   Osteomalacia describes the combination of clinical, biochemical, radiographic and histological abnormalities in adults which result from severe deficiency of vitamin D. In affected bones there is a defect in the proportion of matrix that is mineralised and bone histology is characterised by broadened osteoid seams.   Radiographically there may be characteristic pseudofractures or Looser's zones.   Clinically the syndrome comprises psychological changes, typically depression, neuromuscular changes in the form of a proximal neuromyopathy, generalised pains of uncertain origin but possibly from bone, and fractures following minimal trauma.   Although low plasma 25(OH)vitamin D concentrations on their own are not sufficient to diagnose osteomalacia, plasma 25(OH)vitamin D concentrations less than 4 µg/l (10nmol/l) are seen in adults with osteomalacia.

3.4.2.2 *Rickets*   Rickets occurs after prolonged deficiency of vitamin D during periods of bone growth when an excess of unmineralised osteoid results in a low mineral to bone matrix ratio. Clinically the child is miserable and apathetic and in pain. In severe cases the gait is waddling with bow legs or knock knees. The wrists, ankles and costo-chondral junctions are thickened.   Radiologically the epiphyses show flaring and cupping with widening of the cartilaginous growth plates. Plasma 25(OH)vitamin D concentrations below 8 µg/l (20nmol/l) are seen in children with rickets.

3.4.2.3 *Vitamin D deficiency*   Deficiency of vitamin D, which is less severe than that presenting as osteomalacia or rickets, may also increase the risk of bone disorder.   The clinical presentation may not be distinctive of metabolic bone disorder and is often confounded by multiple nutrient deficiencies, or other influences. Further, non-metabolic mechanisms may account for changes in bone associated with vitamin D insufficiency. For example, the muscle dysfunction which accompanies vitamin D insufficiency may lead to involution by decreasing the strain forces on bone. The response to vitamin therapy in osteomalacia and rickets can be speedy and dramatic. The response to more minor degrees of vitamin D deficiency is usually less overt and, especially in very old people, multiply confounded by other factors[42].

3.5 The assessment of bone health

3.5.1 *Fracture rate*   An important effect of osteoporosis is fracture following minimal trauma. However, fracture is not always clinically apparent, even to the affected individual. The commonest fractures early after the menopause are of the vertebrae, but a substantial proportion pass unrecognised and are only obvious at a later date from radiological examination or as a presumed cause of loss of height. Vertebral fracture cannot therefore be used as a reliable outcome marker for bone health. The other common sites for fracture in older people are the hip and the wrist, where few pass undiagnosed. Recent trials of supplementation with calcium and/or vitamin D confirm that hip fracture rate can be used as an outcome[43,44]. Prospective studies to examine the effect of interventions have only been done in groups of elderly participants aged at least 75 years and over by which age hip fracture incidence is high enough to make studies feasible. This means that there are no data from intervention trials which use hip fracture as the outcome marker in younger postmenopausal women.

3.5.2   *Physical measurements*   In most studies, interventions designed to influence bone status use intermediate outcome measures, the dimensions, mass or mineralisation of the bones, levels of chemical markers of bone metabolism, and bone biopsies. The traditional technique for examining bones is by x-ray. This can show extremes of loss of bone mass with loss of opacity, but this methodology does not discriminate adequately for measuring smaller changes because approximately 30 per cent of skeletal mass has to be lost before x-ray changes are apparent. Assessment of the trabecular structure in the neck of the femur (Singh index) is sometimes used. X-rays are also relatively insensitive in diagnosing vitamin D deficiency in adults and in distinguishing the bony changes of hyperparathyroidism.

3.5.3   Several techniques are available for the assessment of bone mass. Dual energy X-ray absorptiometry (DXA) assesses bone mineral at both axial and appendicular sites, has high reproducibility, and uses low doses of radiation. Sources of error, especially in assessing the spine occur due to the formation of osteophytes in spondylosis and also from calcification of the aorta. Single energy X-ray absorptiometry (SXA) enables measurements only at appendicular sites, such as the forearm. Earlier versions of these techniques, single photon absorptiometry and dual photon absorptiometry, used photons from gamma emitting sources. Quantitative computer tomography enables differential measurement of cortical and trabecular bone in the spine or peripheral skeleton, but the equipment is expensive and the radiation dose is relatively high. Finally, ultrasonic measurements of bone at heel and knee are being evaluated for their reliability in assessing bone. This technique uses a non-ionising radiation, is portable and relatively cheap, but not yet adequately validated for routine use.

3.5.4   Bone mineral mass is a major determinant of risk of future fracture. After linear growth has ceased, whole body bone mineral content (BMC) continues to increase through an increase in bone mineral density (BMD) and possibly some degree of apposition. The rate of increase and its duration vary between individuals and between sexes; peak bone mass occurs at different times in different parts of the body. In adults aged over 40 years at the time of measurement, it reflects the combined effect of achieved peak bone mass diminished by subsequent bone loss. Several prospective studies have shown an increasing gradient of risk of fracture with decrease in both BMC and in BMD. It has been calculated that a reduction of one standard deviation of femoral bone mass below the mean normal value (age related) give a relative risk of fracture of

2.6[45]. Further cohort studies suggest that women over 65 years with a BMD in the lowest quarter of the distribution, after age adjustment, have a risk of hip fracture 8.5 times that of women with BMD in the highest quarter[46]. Although BMC and BMD are powerful predictors of fracture risk within populations, they do not explain differences in fracture incidence between populations. The BMC and BMD of Gambian women are similar to or lower than those of white women and lower than those of black women in North America, but both black populations have lower fracture rates than white American women[47]. Japanese women have both lower BMC and lower fracture rates than white American women[48].

3.5.5   Bone mineral density, as measured by DXA and related techniques, is an areal measurement, representing the amount of mineral within the bone envelope per unit area scanned[49]. It is not a measure of the volumetric density either of the entire bone or of the mineralised tissue within the bone. Similarly, the measured BMC is the mass of mineral within the scanned bone envelope. As a consequence, both BMC and BMD are influenced by the size, shape and orientation of the bone, and can provide no information about internal structure. The interplay of bone mineral measurements, skeletal size and lifestyle factors such as dietary intake and physical activity needs careful consideration when interpreting observational studies[50]. This limits the usefulness of cross-sectional studies and meta-analyses of epidemiological data in examining the relationships between nutrition and bone health, unless steps are taken to minimise the confounding influence of size. Similar considerations are required when comparing individuals and groups of different size, such as children growing at different rates[51,52] or representatives of different ethnic groups[53,54]. In this report, evidence relying on the measurement of bone mineral has been taken from longitudinal and intervention studies wherever possible.

3.5.6   *Biochemical markers and calciotropic hormones*   Bone loss reflects excess bone resorption over bone formation, but both of these processes may be increased in osteoporosis. It has been suggested that the rate of bone loss can be predicted by assessing bone turnover through blood and/or urinary markers that are specific to bone formation and resorption and many have been proposed. Plasma levels of osteocalcin, procollagen carboxy peptide and procollagen amino peptide, and bone specific alkaline phosphatase are validated indices of bone formation reflecting activity of osteoblasts. More recently, urinary pyridinoline crosslinks and related peptides, which are sensitive and specific markers of bone resorption, have become widely used[55]. Urinary hydroxyproline and fasting urinary calcium/creatinine ratios, used in the past, were found to be poor indices of resorption. There is much interest in whether the predictive value in respect of future bone loss is improved if markers both of formation and of resorption are assessed simultaneously to reflect the dynamic process of bone turnover.

4.   Dietary Reference Values

4.1   Background

4.1.1   Nutrient intakes must be sufficient to meet metabolic demands and to allow for growth in the young. There are considerable variations between individuals and in individuals over time. The factors influencing this variation include age, genetic make-up, body size and state of health, as well as others. The composition of the diet is also important because of interactions between different nutrients which affect the degree to which an individual nutrient is absorbed in the gut and its metabolic availability. Because of this heterogeneity, diets of populations are assessed for adequacy on a group basis in order to take account of day to day dietary variations by measuring intakes over several days, as well as of external factors such as season of the year. On this basis, most countries have declared yardstick values for dietary guidance and planning (Annex 1). In the UK these values are called Dietary Reference Values (DRVs) and they are used to assist in interpreting dietary intake information in individuals and groups.

4.1.2   Each nutrient is considered individually and all the available information is taken into account in setting the three values which are described below. The estimates of requirements for nutrients have been based on information from:

- the intakes of a nutrient needed to maintain a given circulating level or degree of enzyme saturation or tissue concentration;

- the intakes of a nutrient by individuals and by groups which are associated with the absence of any signs of deficiency diseases;

- the intakes of a nutrient needed to maintain balance noting that the period over which such balance needs to be measured differs for different nutrients, and between individuals;

- the intakes of a nutrient needed to cure clinical signs of deficiency;

- the intakes of a nutrient associated with an appropriate biological marker of structural and functional adequacy.

4.2   Dietary Reference Values

4.2.1   Dietary Reference Values for energy and nutrients were most recently set for the UK in 1991[17]**. They define the range of estimated dietary requirements

---

** This publication was reprinted with textual corrections in 1994; at the same time, in the section on fluoride, the safe intake levels were amended [56].

in different groups of individuals. They take account of the biological variation between individuals which determines differing energy and nutrient needs to meet specified criteria. Normal metabolic needs for healthy individuals, such as the needs for growth, are taken into account, although the DRVs make no allowances for the different energy and nutrient needs imposed by diseases. DRVs used for food labelling purposes are specified separately and are common throughout the European Union[57].

4.2.2   For most nutrients the DRVs comprise three levels of intake: the Estimated Average Requirement (EAR) of a group for that nutrient; the Reference Nutrient Intake (RNI) which is sufficient to cover the needs of nearly all the population group and the Lower Reference Nutrient Intake (LRNI) sufficient only for those with the lowest requirements. In developing these values, it has generally been assumed that the distribution of requirements for a nutrient is normal. Even when the distribution of intakes in a population is constant, the individuals comprising the extremes are likely to vary from day to day. In addition there is, for most nutrients, only scant information about homeostatic mechanisms including changes in absorption which could influence dietary requirement. It is assumed that there is some relationship between nutrient requirement and spontaneous intake, for instance for energy requirements because of body size. Thus, in a group of individuals with a mean intake at the RNI level, the likelihood of a significant number of individuals not meeting their requirements is very small. The concepts on which the DRVs were based have been described more fully in the original report. Relevant paragraphs have been reproduced in Annex 2.

4.2.3   In many cases, the data about nutrient requirements were only adequate to set a RNI, as a level likely to meet the needs of virtually everyone in the specified population group e.g. vitamin D. For energy it is important to consume neither insufficient nor excess and only an EAR was given. Where there were insufficient data to set DRVs but the function of the nutrient (pantothenic acid, biotin, vitamin E, vitamin K, manganese, molybdenum, chromium and fluoride) is important, values for an intake, or range of intakes, were estimated as sufficient to meet the need of all individuals but not so high as to cause adverse effects. This was called a "safe intake", at which level there was judged to be minimal risk of undesirable effects from too low or high an intake in any individual.

(i)   *Estimated Average Requirement* (EAR) - The estimate of the average dietary requirement for food energy or a nutrient.

(ii)   *Reference Nutrient Intake* (RNI) - The amount of a nutrient that is enough for almost every individual, even someone who has high needs for the nutrient in the distribution of individual requirements. Notionally it represents a value 2 standard deviations above the EAR. The level of intake is, therefore, considerably higher than most people need and individuals consuming the RNI are most unlikely to be deficient. If the average intake of a group is at the level of the RNI, then the risk of deficiency in the group would be expected to be very low.

16

(iii)   *Lower Reference Nutrient Intake* (LRNI) - A nutrient intake level notionally representing 2 standard deviations below the EAR. This amount is enough for only the small number of people who have the lowest needs. People habitually having intakes less than the LRNI will almost certainly be deficient.

4.2.4   The COMA Subgroup on Bone Health was asked to review the DRVs for calcium and vitamin D. It has not re-assessed in detail the data on which the DRVs for these nutrients were based in 1991 by the COMA Working Party on Dietary Reference Values. Rather, it has considered whether the DRVs should be changed in the light of more recently available information. Brief mention is made about other nutrients which might plausibly have an influence on bone health (para 7.2). The review by this Subgroup has not considered these nutrients in the same detail.

4.3   Dietary Reference Values for calcium

4.3.1   *The UK DRVs for calcium* set in 1991 (Table 4.1) were derived by calculating factorially from the needs for calcium for growth and for maintenance of bone mineralisation. Allowances were made for incomplete absorption and obligatory calcium losses. Markers of bone status were not used as criteria, nor any aspect of bone health, in setting the DRVs. A comparison with the national statements concerning population nutrient intakes for calcium from other countries is at Annex 1. The UK term "Reference Nutrient Intake" is matched by other terminologies but all implying a value which is likely to provide for the nutrient needs of almost all of the population (para 4.2).

Table 4.1 UK Dietary Reference Values for calcium (mg/d(mmol/d))[17]

| | POPULATION GROUPS | | | | | | |
	0-12 months	1-3 years	4-6 years	7-10 years	11-18 yrs M/F	19+ years	Lactation
RNI	525 (13.1)	350 (8.8)	450 (11.3)	550 (13.8)	1000/800 (25.0/20.0)	700 (17.5)	+550 (+14.3)
LRNI	240 (6.0)	200 (5.0)	275 (6.9)	325 (8.1)	480/450 (12.0/11.3)	400 (10.0)	

Notes: RNI = Reference Nutrient Intake   M = Male
           LRNI = Lower Reference Nutrient Intake   F = Female

4.3.2   *USA National Institutes of Health Consensus Development Panel*   In 1994, the USA National Institutes of Health convened a consensus conference with other USA professional, scientific and consumer bodies to attempt to define an optimal calcium intake at different ages[15]. In reaching conclusions, the conference rejected previous approaches in favour of "optimal function" as a basis for their calculations. Thus, accepting the relationship between bone mineral content/density and fracture risk, thresholds were determined for intakes of calcium, above which there would be no additional increase in BMC/BMD. On this basis, values were published as representing "Optimal Calcium Requirements" for different population groups (Table 4.2). These intake levels were all higher than the respective USA Recommended Dietary Allowance and UK RNI values (Annex 1).

Table 4.2 Optional calcium requirements recommended by the USA National Institutes of Health Concensus Panel 1994[15]

POPULATION GROUP	"Optimal Daily Intake" of calcium (mg)
0-6 months	400
6-12 months	600
1-5 years	800
6-10 years	800-1200
11-24 years	1200-1500
Men	
25-65 years	1000
Over 65 years	1500
Women	
25-50 years	1000
Over 50 years (postmenopausal)	
On oestrogens	1000
Not on oestrogens	1500
Over 65 years	1500
Pregnant or lactating	1200-1500

4.3.3   The NIH Consensus Panel defined optimal calcium intake as the levels of consumption that are necessary (a) to maximise peak adult bone mass, (b) to maintain adult bone mass, and (c) to minimise bone loss in the later years. Studies related to calcium intake and its effects on calcium balance, bone mass and the prevention of osteoporosis were reviewed.   The report gave insufficient information to evaluate the basis of the figures proposed for different age groups. No evidence was given to demonstrate that the experimental measures used have been validated as predictors of the desired functional end-points. In addition, the data presented were not compatible with the calculation of an EAR or RNI for the setting of Dietary Reference Values using the model adopted by the UK Committee on Medical Aspects of Food and Nutrition Policy. The Subgroup on Bone Health reviewed the evidence presented by the NIH Consensus Panel and could find no scientific justification to adopt their recommendations at this stage. It would be important to ensure that there would be no associated adverse effects if the population intakes of calcium were to increase to the levels suggested by the Consensus Panel.

4.3.4   *Recommendations for calcium intake from other countries*   Annex 1 gives the Dietary Reference Values for calcium for population groups in different countries. The basis for the European Union estimates for Population Reference Intakes and also for the French recommendations were similar to that used by the UK, namely factorial and takes account of the requirements for growth, with allowances for obligatory losses and varying absorption[57,58]. The Australian and New Zealand Recommended Dietary Intakes are based on values calculated to provide enough absorbed calcium to meet obligatory losses, needs for growth and an additional allowance at 200mg calcium per day for women over 50 years designed, in their view, to recognise the potential role of calcium in the prevention of postmenopausal osteoporosis[59,60].

4.3.5   *Dietary Reference Intakes for the USA and Canada*   The USA in reviewing its equivalent of the UK DRVs, formerly used a philosophy similar to the UK's to derive its values for calcium factorially[16]. The Food and Nutrition

Board of the Institutes of Medicine, with the involvement of Health Canada, has recently undertaken a re-evaluation of Dietary Reference Intakes for the United States and Canada[61]. The report of their findings for calcium, phosphorus, magnesium, vitamin D and fluoride was made public in August 1997. This was after the final meeting of the Subgroup on Bone Health and was not included in their deliberations. The general model adopted for the re-evaluation of each nutrient by the Food and Nutrition Board was similar to that of the UK DRV Committee. Evidence was reviewed for each nutrient (a) to establish whether an estimated average requirement (EAR) could be defined based on a specified indicator of adequacy, (b) if so, to calculate a recommended dietary allowance (RDA) from EAR+2sd (equivalent to the UK RNI) and (c) if not, to estimate an adequate intake (AI) that appears to be sufficient to sustain a defined nutritional state. In addition, hazard identification and risk assessments were made in order to set a tolerable upper intake level (UL).

4.3.6   The Food and Nutrition Board after reviewing the data felt able only to propose AI values for calcium because of the lack of scientific evidence. The AI was defined as an experimentally derived approximate group mean intake value, based on a limited selection of calcium intakes that appear to support maximal calcium retention. The assumption was made that maximal calcium retention may reduce the risk of fracture secondary to osteopenia or osteoporosis. Supporting evidence was taken from studies relating calcium intake to calcium biochemistry, bone mineral density and fracture rates. A tolerable upper intake level was set at 2000mg Ca/day for adults, at 2500mg Ca/day for children, adolescents, pregnant and lactating women and adults >70y[61].

4.4   Dietary Reference Values for vitamin D

4.4.1   *The UK DRVs for vitamin D*   In the UK, Reference Nutrient Intake values only are given for vitamin D and only for limited age groups. The RNI for infants up to 6 months is 8.5 µg/day, from 6 months to the end of 3 years it is 7 µg/day, and for pregnant and lactating women and for people aged 65 years or over it is 10 µg/day. Between ages 4 and 64 years no RNI is set; it is assumed that skin synthesis of vitamin D will generally ensure adequacy which depends on regular exposure to summer sunlight. Within this group are individuals who are at risk of vitamin D deficiency and who require dietary vitamin D if they are to maintain adequate status, for example where exposure to sunlight is restricted by extensive concealment with clothing or if the person does not go out of doors, or if the skin is pigmented (para 6.2.14) especially if their diet excludes meat and oily fish. For these an RNI of 10 µg/day is set.

4.4.2   *Recommendations for vitamin D intake from other countries*   Annex 1 gives the Dietary Reference Values for vitamin D for population groups in different countries. The values for most countries were based on the dietary intake needed to maintain the circulating plasma 25(OH)vitamin D concentration at normal levels in the absence of exposure to sunlight[57,58,62]. The US RDA was also set on the basis of the dietary requirement when there is insufficient exposure to sunlight with additional allowances for times when there is calcium deposition in bones during childhood, and in the fetus or infant during pregnancy and

19

lactation[16]. The Australian Recommended Dietary Intakes assumed that there would be adequate exposure to sunlight and a dietary source is only indicated in exceptional circumstances and stated that housebound people might benefit from an oral intake of 10 μg/day of vitamin D[59].

4.4.3   *Dietary Reference Intakes for vitamin D for the USA and Canada* The principles underlying the 1997 revision of the USA Reference Dietary Intakes have been described earlier (para 4.3.5). As for calcium (para 4.3.5.2), the Food and Nutrition Board felt able only to propose an AI value for each population group for vitamin D, which was defined as the group mean intake value that appears to be needed to maintain, in a defined group of individuals with limited but uncertain sun exposure and stores, plasma 25(OH)vitamin D above a defined amount[61]. The latter is that concentration below which vitamin D deficiency rickets or osteomalacia occurs. The intake value was rounded to the nearest 50IU (1.25 μg) and then doubled as a safety factor to cover the needs of all, regardless of exposure to sun (Annex 1). A tolerable upper intake level was set at 25 μg/day for infants and 50 μg/day for all other population groups.

5. Reassessment of the Dietary Reference Values for calcium

5.1 Conclusions

5.1.1 No revision of the calcium DRVs for infants is proposed; there have been no relevant data since 1991 (para 5.4.1).

5.1.2 After reviewing the evidence, it was felt that the available data were not sufficient to warrant revising the DRVs for calcium for children and adolescents. More studies with long term follow-up are required (para 5.4.6).

5.1.3 The RNI for calcium for adults, except lactating women, is 700mg/d. Although there has been much debate about whether it represents an adequate intake, the data on which to base proposals for an increase are few. In particular, studies with long term follow-up and using clinical outcome measures are needed. There is evidence that calcium intakes below the current LRNI of 400mg/d might not be compatible with good bone health. The Subgroup therefore did not propose changes to the current DRVs for calcium (para 5.4.12.2).

5.1.4 The factors taken into account by the DRV Panel in 1991 in deciding that the RNI for calcium during pregnancy should be the same as for adults who are not pregnant were reviewed and confirmed. The Subgroup found no basis on which to recommend otherwise (para 5.4.13).

5.1.5 The UK RNI for calcium during lactation includes an additional 550mg derived factorially. Recent data suggest that this increment might not be necessary. The Subgroup considered it prudent to await further data before deciding whether to revise this increment (para 5.4.14).

5.2 Metabolism of calcium and bone status

5.2.1 More than 99 per cent of the body's calcium resides in the skeleton, mainly as crystalline hydroxyapatite. The remaining one per cent is in tissues and fluids, where it is essential for maintaining biomembrane integrity and permeability (which is important for normal neuromuscular function), inter-cellular and intra-cellular signalling and enzyme regulation. During childhood and young adulthood, bone mineral content increases to a peak at about 30 years of age, after which it declines slowly. It is important to ensure that the calcium needs of the growing skeleton are met: at birth the total body calcium is 25g and in adulthood it is about 1000g.

5.2.2 *Calcium absorption from foods*   Calcium absorption, which is modulated by vitamin D (para 6.2.2), occurs predominantly in the jejunum, and also in the ileum and colon. It can be measured by a variety of techniques, the most accurate is isotopic labelling[63]. As calcium intakes increase, the active mechanism becomes saturated and any further calcium absorption occurs by passive diffusion. The net result is an increase in the absolute amount of absorbed calcium with increasing intake but a decrease in fractional absorption. Increased fractional calcium absorption has been demonstrated during the months August to October when compared with March to May[64]. These mechanisms may in part account for the different results from absorption and calcium balance studies on populations with higher or lower customary intakes of calcium.

5.2.3   Most of the calcium in foods forms complexes with other dietary constituents. Gastric acid secretions assist the solubility of calcium salts. Thus, reduced acid secretion, which is more common in older people, reduces the absorption of calcium. The calcium in milk is better absorbed than that from most other sources. Calcium from breast milk is absorbed more efficiently than calcium from cows' milk or infant formula[17]. Particular dietary components such as oxalate, phytate, protein and other substances are more likely to bind the calcium in large molecular complexes. A diet of cereals which is rich in many of these substances should theoretically decrease calcium absorption by binding calcium in the small intestine, but the results have been unpredictable in studies using test diets[63]. Diets rich in bran are generally associated with reduced calcium absorption[65] but it is still unknown to what extent hydrolysis in the lower intestine can compensate for high intakes of phytate in humans through the release of bound calcium and subsequent absorption. There may also be competition with other divalent cations such as Fe^{++} which may reduce the absorption of Ca^{++}. Other dietary components such as fat, phosphate, magnesium, caffeine and non-starch polysaccharide (with the exception of large amounts) have not been found to affect the overall retention or excretion of calcium significantly although they can have short term effects on absorption and excretion rates[66]. Diet composition, for example sodium and high dietary protein intakes have also been associated with increased urinary calcium[67].

5.2.4   Individuals demonstrate great physiological adaptability in their absorption, excretion and metabolic use of dietary calcium. For example, during periods of growth when the biological requirement is high[68], calcium conservation mechanisms become more efficient if calcium intake is low[69]. There are also physiological changes in calcium and bone metabolism during pregnancy and lactation to meet the increased demand for calcium (para 5.4.13, 5.4.14). Little is known about whether the adaptive response is limited by factors such as age, oestrogen status and exposure to high or low calcium intakes early in life and nothing is known about the range of inter-individual variability in the capacity to adapt to low calcium diets. The major determinant of calcium homeostasis appears to be the plasma level of ionised calcium, sustained in part by the mobilisation and deposition of skeletal calcium (see para 3.3.3). This immediate response to a diminishing calcium supply is thought to precede adaptation to increase calcium absorption and decrease calcium excretion. In adults, adaptation to a change in diet can be very slow; adult men introduced to a diet containing half the amount of calcium than their customary diet took several months to regain calcium balance[70]. This is an important qualifying factor in using balance studies to assess dietary calcium needs (para 4.1.2). These variations in bioefficacy need to be accommodated within any consideration of the nutrient adequacy of the diet.

5.2.5   *Adverse effects of high calcium intakes*   Body calcium metabolism is under such close homeostatic control that an excessive accumulation in blood or tissues from overconsumption is virtually unknown. Life-threatening calcium toxicity is rare but is evident in case reports of "milk-alkali syndrome", presenting with hypercalcaemia, metabolic alkalosis and renal failure, caused by the consumption of very high amounts of both calcium and alkali that can lead to promotion of calcium retention[71]. The Food and Nutrition Board of the USA National Institutes of Medicine set an upper tolerable intake level of 2000mg/day for most adults and 2500mg/day for other population groups (para 4.3.6)[61]. High dietary calcium intakes appear to decrease the risk of symptomatic kidney stones but use of calcium supplements may increase the risk[71,72]. High calcium diets can influence the bioefficacy of other minerals. Calcium inhibits iron absorption and studies in humans suggest that high-calcium diets affect zinc metabolism but the exact mechanism is not known[71,73].

5.3   Dietary Reference Values for calcium: a review of the evidence

5.3.1   The DRVs for calcium were set in the UK in 1991[17]. The basis for the values chosen was factorial calculations, which took account of that amount of calcium needed to cover involuntary calcium losses as well as increments for growth in childhood. COMA did not consider that bone status was sensitive as a marker of nutritional status in regard to calcium. It rejected all of the measures of bone health, fracture, BMC, BMD, and bone biochemical markers because of the difficulties of relating calcium status to long term functional outcome and because of the several confounding factors influencing bone health. They concluded that there were no markers of bone health that were useful as indicators of calcium nutritional status.

5.3.2   In reviewing the DRV for this report the Subgroup looked for evidence of a benefit of higher intakes than the current RNI, wherever possible from longitudinal and intervention trials.

5.4   Dietary Reference Values for calcium for different population groups

5.4.1   *Infants*

RNI 525mg/d(13.1mmol); LRNI 240 mg/d(6.0mmol)

Breastmilk calcium levels decline after the first 12 weeks of lactation. The levels vary between individuals and between communities. Communities with low dietary calcium intakes may have low breastmilk calcium levels, but this is not inevitable[74]. Supplementation studies have shown that breast milk calcium concentrations are not responsive to an increase in calcium intake by lactating mothers[75,76]. In this country, an average calcium intake for breastfed infants is

250mg/day[77], and it is assumed that 55-60 per cent is absorbed. Only about 40 per cent of the calcium in cows' milk-based formulas is absorbed, so the calcium level in these products is set higher to compensate.

In conclusion:

No revision of the calcium DRVs for infants is proposed; there have been no relevant data since 1991 (conclusion 5.1.1).

5.4.2   *Children and adolescents*
> *1-3 years: RNI 350mg/d(8.8mmol); LRNI 200mg/d(5.0mmol)*
> *4-6 years: RNI 450mg/d(11.3mmol); LRNI 275mg/d(6.9mmol)*
> *7-10 years: RNI 550mg/d(13.8mmol); LRNI 325mg/d(8.1mmol)*
> *11-18 years: RNI male 1000mg/d(25.0mmol);*
> *female 800mg/d(20.0mmol);*
> *LRNI male 480mg/d(12.0mmol); female 450mg/d(11.3mmol)*

5.4.3   Children need to absorb 70-150mg calcium per day for growth and bone mineralisation. During adolescence bone growth is considerable, and greater for boys. This requires a daily absorbed amount of calcium of at least 250mg for girls and 300mg for boys, and it can be higher. It is agreed that it is important to meet these requirements in order to achieve a peak bone mass which reflects the genetic potential of each individual[78]. A high peak bone mass helps to ensure that as age related bone loss occurs it does not lead to a level of bone mass so low that the risk of fracture increases in old age. It has been suggested that low calcium intakes may contribute to stunting (linear growth retardation), which is the most common disorder of skeletal growth on a world scale. The aetiology of stunting is complex and is generally considered a manifestation of chronic malnutrition[79]. It is plausible that low intakes of calcium might be important in determining poor growth performance, but data are lacking[80].

5.4.4   Several recent supplementation studies of children and adolescents have observed increases in BMC and BMD of 2-6 per cent in response to supplementation with calcium salts (Table 5.1a, 5.1b)[81,82,83,84,85,86].   In general, this has not been associated with alterations in skeletal size although increases at the lumbar spine have been reported[83,85]. There is no obvious relationship between the magnitude of the increase in bone mineral achieved in the different studies and the customary calcium intake of the study group or the level of calcium supplementation used[78]. It is possible that the response may be greater in, or limited to, children with lower calcium intake[85] or who are at specific stages of development[81,84,86] but the data are not consistent[82,83,84,87].

5.4.5   Few studies have examined the mechanism underlying the response to changes in calcium intake or have investigated long term benefit, but several are in progress. There is evidence that the increase in bone mineral appears early in the supplementation period with little additional effect thereafter[81,86], that it is associated with a decrease in bone formation as demonstrated by plasma osteocalcin concentrations[81] and that it disappears on withdrawal of the

Table 5.1a Calcium supplementation studies in children and adolescents (all randomised controlled trials) (see also Table 5.1b)

Country and pubertal status	Age on entry to the study (years)	Sex	Number in group Suppl	Number in group Unsuppl	Calcium intake (mg/d) (mean) Diet	Calcium intake (mg/d) (mean) Suppl	Duration of supple-mentation (months)	Osteocalcin levels in blood (bone turnover)	Bone effect (see also table 5.1b)	Follow-up†
Pre-puberty USA Johnston et al 1992 [81] Slemenda et al 1997 [96]	7	M + F	22*	22*	900	1000 CCM	36	Reduced	+	0
China Lee et al 1994 [82] Lee et al 1997 [97]	7	M + F	79	83	280	300 CaCo$_3$	18	nm	+	0
Hong Kong Lee et al 1995 [83] Lee et al 1996 [98]	7	M + F	44	40	570	300 CaCo$_3$	18	nm	+	0
Switzerland Bonjour et al 1997 [85]	8 8	F F	36 31	36 41	<880 >880	850 Caphos 850 Caphos	12 12	nm nm	+ 0	+ 0
Peri-and post-puberty USA Johnston et al 1992 [81] Slemenda et al 1997 [96]	11	M + F	23*	23*	900	1000 CCM	36	No change	0	0
USA Lloyd et al 1993 [99] Lloyd et al 1996 [84]	12	F	48	46	960	500 CCM	18,24	nm	+	nr
USA Andon et al 1994 [100]	11	F	120	128	880	500/1000 CCM	6	nm	+	nr
Pre-peri and post-puberty Australia Nowson et al 1997 $ [86]	14	F	42*	42*	730	1000 CLG	6,12,18	nm	+**	nr
The Gambia Dibba et al 1997 [87]	10	M + F	80	80	350	714 CaCO$_3$	12	nm	+	nr

Notes:
M = male; F = female
CCM = calcium citrate malate
Caphos = calcium phosphate extracted from milk
CLG = calcium lactate gluconate
nm = not measured
nr = not reported

+ = an increase in bone mineral
$ = no evidence of an effect of pubertal status
0 = no effect
† difference between groups several months after stopping the supplement
* twin studies
** effect confined to first 6 months with no further effect by 18 months

25

Table 5.1b Calcium supplementation studies in children and adolescents: magnitude of the bone effect at different skeletal sites (see also Table 5.1a) (results presented here have been reworked from the original data)

Country and pubertal status	Bone mineral content Skeletal site				Bone mineral density Skeletal site				Bone area Skeletal site				Height
	TB	RS	LS	FN	TB	RS	LS	FN	TB	RS	LS	FN	
Pre-puberty USA Johnston et al 1992 [81]	nm	nr	nr	nr	nm	+5.1†	+2.8†	+1.2	nm	nr	nr	nr	0
China Lee et al 1994 [82]	nm	+2.3*	nm	nm	nm	+3.2**	nm	nm	nm	-0.7	nm	nm	0
Hong Kong Lee et al 1995 [83]	nm	+0.9	+4.7*	+0.8	nm	+1.7	+3.7	-0.6	nm	-1.0	+2.5*	+1.6	0
Peri- and post-puberty USA Johnston et al 1992 [81]	nm	nr	nr	nr	nm	-0.1	-1.0	-0.4	nm	nr	nr	nr	0
USA Lloyd et al 1993 at 18 mth [99]	+2.0	nm	+4.7	nm	+1.3*	nm	+2.9*	nm	-3.6	nm	+0.5	nm	0
USA Lloyd et al 1996 at 24 mth [84]	+4.6*	nm	+7.8*	nm	+2.1**	nm	+4.1*	nm	+1.7	nm	+2.5	nm	0
USA Andon et al 1994 [100]	+1.1/+2.2*	nm	nm	nm	nr	nm	nm	nm	nr	nm	nm	nm	nm
Pre-, peri- and post-puberty combined USA Johnston et al 1992 [81]	nm	nr	nr	nr	nm	+2.5†	+0.7	+0.4	nm	-0.3	-1.7	+3.9	0
Australia Nowson et al 1997*** [86]	nm	nm	nr	nr	nm	nm	+1.5**	+1.1	nm	nm	0	nr	0
The Gambia Dibba et al 1997 [87]	nm	+4.0*	nm	nm	nm	+5.1**	nm	nm	nm	-1.0	nm	nm	0

Notes: nm = not measured; nr = not reported; 0 = no effect

Data are per cent increase in supplemented group minus per cent increase in placebo group

† 95% confidence interval did not include zero;

* p<0.05; ** p <0.01; no other differences were statistically significant

*** effect confined to first 6 months

TB = total body; RS = radius shaft; LS = lumbar spine; FN = femoral neck. (Other sites were monitored in individual studies, e.g. wrist, pelvis, Ward's triangle, trochanter - not presented in this table)

26

supplement[82,83,88]. This pattern suggests that the increase is due to the bone-remodelling transient (para 3.3.3), in which a decrease in bone turnover is accompanied by a reversible, incremental increase in bone mineral due to reduced numbers of resorption cavities on bone surfaces[28]. There are no data to determine whether an increase in bone mineral associated with decreased bone formation or turnover represents a benefit for growing children nor whether it results in an increase in peak bone mass in adulthood.

5.4.6   *Milk and bone health*   Retrospective and ecological studies reporting a link between high calcium intake in childhood and decreased risk of osteoporosis in later life[89] have generally quantified milk intake[90] but many have failed to take account of confounding factors such as physical activity[91]. Recent evidence suggests that milk may exert an anabolic effect on the growing skeleton that is different from that of calcium salts alone, possibly as a result of the associated increase in protein intake[92]. Increases in bone mineral have also been observed after supplementation with milk and dairy products[92,93]. In the longer term, a study of Welsh children who had participated in a two-year milk supplementation trial at age 7-9 years found no evidence of increased bone mineral at 20-23 years[94]. Between country comparisons show a positive association between higher customary calcium intakes generally due to high intakes of milk and higher rates of hip fracture in older age[95] but these correlations are confounded by several factors including particularly differences in the levels of physical activity and vitamin D status between the populations being compared.

In conclusion:

After reviewing the evidence, it was felt that the available data were not sufficient to warrant revising the DRVs for calcium for children and adolescents. More studies with long term follow-up are required (conclusion 5.1.2).

5.4.7   *Adults*
RNI 700mg/d(17.5mmol); LRNI 400mg/d(10.0mmol)

5.4.8   *Younger adults*   Once maximum height has been reached, there is a limited increase in bone mass, of around 5 per cent of the total, before peak bone mass is attained. Bone remodelling continues to renew, reshape and repair the bones and there is a small but significant periosteal apposition as the long bones get broader throughout life. From about age 35-40 years, bone mineral is lost at an average rate of 0.3-0.4 per cent of bone mass per year.

5.4.9   *Peri- and postmenopausal women*   The menopause is defined as the cessation of menses which marks failure of the ovarian function to secrete the sex hormones, oestrogen and progesterone. In the peri- and early postmenopausal period there is sparse evidence to link bone loss with customary calcium intake, or little to support widespread pharmacological calcium supplementation. In studies which have included both early postmenopausal and older women, calcium supplementation appears to have had little effect on BMD in women who

Table 5.2 Calcium supplementation in healthy early postmenopausal women: controlled studies of the magnitude of the effect on bone loss (results presented here have been reworked from the original data)

Country	Mean age (years)	Years since menopause	Number in group		Study design		Calcium intake (mg/d) (mean)		Duration of supplementation (years)	Bone site	Bone loss		Effect of suppl on bone loss	Statistical significance
			Suppl	Unsuppl	R	P	Diet	Supplement			Suppl	Unsuppl		
Netherlands Elders et al 1994 [105]	50	Peri + PM	104	61	✓	X	1040	2000 / 1000	3	LS / MC	Y / Y	Y / Y	0 / +	NS / <0.01
USA Aloia et al 1994 [106]	52	0.5-6	34	36	✓	✓	480	1200*	2.9	LS / FN / W / Troc / RP / WB	Y / Y / Y / N / Y	Y / Y / Y / Y / N / Y	0 / + / 0 / 0 / 0 / +	NS / 0.03 / NS / NS / NS / 0.006
USA Dawson-Hughes et al 1990 [101]	55	3 (<5)	53	16	✓	✓	approx 400	500	2	LS / FN / RP	Y / N / N	Y / N / N	0 / 0 / (+)	NS / NS / NS
USA Ettinger et al 1987 [102]	52	0.5-3	36	19	X	X	660	1000	2	LS / RP / MC	Y / (Y) / Y	Y / Y / Y	0 / 0 / 0	NS / NS / NS
Denmark Riis et al 1987 [107]	50	1.5	14	11	✓	✓	nm	2000	2	LS / WB / FP / FD	Y / Y / Y / Y	Y / Y / Y / Y	0 / (+) / + / 0	NS / NS / <0.05 / NS

Notes: R = randomised; P = placebo controlled; ✓ = yes; X = neither R nor P apply;

Peri = perimenopausal; PM = post menopausal; NS = no statistically significant difference; nm = not measured; * each participant supplemented with calcium to achieve a total daily intake of 1700mg.

Bone site:

LS= lumbar spine; MC = metacarpals; FN = femoral neck (hip); W = Ward's triangle (hip); Troc = trochanter (hip); RP = radius proximal; WB = whole body; FP = forearm proximal; FD = forearm distal

Bone loss:

Y = loss significantly different from 0; (Y) = loss >1% per year but NS;

N = significant bone gain, or no bone loss

Effect of supplementation on bone loss:

+ = reduced bone loss P<0.05; (+) = magnitude of difference in loss >1% per year but P >0.05;

0 = magnitude of difference in loss <1% per year, P >0.05.

are within the first five years after the menopause[101] (Table 5.2). The most effective means of preserving bone mass in early postmenopausal women is through the use of oestrogen replacement therapy[2]. One study has suggested that calcium intake may influence the effect of hormone replacement therapy (HRT) on BMD so that a reduced dose of oestrogen may be required with a higher calcium intake[102]. A recent analysis of HRT trials which compared those in which calcium intake was also increased with those with no dietary modification suggested that the response to HRT may be greater in women who also increase their calcium intake[103]. In this analysis, the average calcium intake of women without dietary modification was 563mg/day. These findings are consistent with data from older women which suggest that a low calcium intake is not compatible with good bone health and that this includes women on HRT. These findings require formal testing[104].

5.4.10   *Older women*

5.4.10.1 *Calcium supplementation trials and bone loss*   In studies of calcium supplementation of women several years after the menopause (both subjects selected from the general population and those with osteoporosis), where significant bone loss was recorded in the control group, calcium supplementation did not prevent some bone loss from occurring. However, in general, women receiving calcium supplements had BMDs that were 1-3 per cent higher than those who did not receive supplements, particularly in regions of the skeleton rich in cortical bone (Table 5.3). Long term studies suggest that any effects of calcium supplementation largely occur in the first 1-2 years[105,108] and that they are mediated by a reduction in bone turnover[109,110]. The role of customary calcium intake is still unclear. In one study[101] the effect on bone was limited to those with daily calcium intakes less than 400mg/day compared with those whose intake was in the range 400-650mg/day. In other studies, any effect of calcium supplementation was not related to the customary dietary intake of calcium.

5.4.10.2 *Calcium supplementation trials and fracture*
(i)   Case-control studies in Britain[122], Australia[123] and Canada[124] have all reported no relationship between calcium intake and risk of hip fracture. In contrast, case-control studies from Hong Kong[125] and Southern Europe[126] suggest an increasing risk of hip fracture with declining calcium intake.

(ii)   Cohort studies on groups of elderly people have also been inconsistent: in Britain[127] and the United States[128] no relationship between calcium intakes and risk of hip fracture was suggested, while a second US study[129] reported a significant increase in hip fracture risk with declining calcium intake. Although these studies differ in the populations selected and several other potential confounding variables for hip fracture risk, their findings are consistent with a threshold for increasing fracture risk below calcium intake around 400-500mg daily. A recent meta-analysis of studies of the relation between calcium intake and fracture risk supported the likelihood, on the basis of observational studies, that a low calcium intake i.e. below the UK LRNI is not compatible with good bone health[130]. Intakes in Hong Kong and certain parts of the United States fall below these levels and it is noteworthy that studies performed in these areas have demonstrated beneficial effects of calcium intake on hip fracture risk.

Table 5.3 Calcium supplementation in women more than 5 years beyond the menopause: controlled studies of the magnitude of the effect on bone loss (results presented here have been reworked from the original data)

Country	Mean age (years)	Years since menopause	Number in group — Suppl	Number in group — Unsuppl	Study design — R	Study design — P	Calcium intake (mg/d) (mean) — Diet	Calcium intake — Supplement	Duration of supplementation (years)	Bone site	Bone loss — Suppl	Bone loss — Unsuppl	Effect of suppl on bone loss	Statistical significance
USA Riggs 1998 [114]	66	16	88	89	✓	✓	710	1600	4*	LS	N	N	0	NS
										FN	N	N	+	<0.05
										WB	N	N	+	<0.05
USA Recker et al 1996 [111]	75(VF)	nr	51	41	✓	✓	450 (<1000)	1200	4.3	RP	N	Y	+	<0.001
	72(NVF)	nr	40	59	✓	✓	410 (<1000)	1200	4.3	RP	N	Y	0	NS
Australia Prince et al 1995 [110]	63	16 (>10)	42	42	✓	✓	800 (<1000)	1000	2	LS	N	N	0	NS
										FN	Y	Y	0	NS
										Troc	N	Y	+	<0.05
										Int	N	Y	+	<0.05
										Ankle	Y	Y	+	<0.05
New Zealand Reid et al 1993 (a) [109] 1995 (b) [108] *(0-2=a, 2-4=b)*	58	9 (>3)	(a) 61 (b) subset 38	(a) 61 (b) subset 40	✓	✓	750	1000	(a) 2 (b) 4	LS	N / N	N / N	0 / 0	NS / NS
										FN	N / Y	Y / Y	+ / 0	0.04 / NS
										W	N / Y	Y / Y	+ / 0	NS / NS
										Troc	Y / N	Y / N	+ / 0	0.04 / NS
										WB	Y / Y	Y / Y	+ / +	0.005 / 0.02
Switzerland Chevalley et al 1994 [112]	72	23	55	25	✓	✓	620	800	1.5	LS	N	N	0	NS
										FN	N	N	(+)	NS
										FP	N	Y	+	<0.05
Hong Kong Lau et al 1992 [113]	75	nr	12	12	✓	✓	260	800	0.8	LS	(Y)	(Y)	(+)	NS
										FN	(Y)	(Y)	(-)	NS
										W	N	N	+	<0.05
										Int	N	Y	+	<0.05
USA Dawson-Hughes et al 1990 [101]	60	13 (>5)	62	33	✓	✓	<400	500	2	LS	N	Y	+	<0.05
										FN	N	Y	+	<0.05
										RP	N	Y	+	<0.05
				53	44			>400	500	2	LS	Y	Y	0	NS
										FN	N	N	0	NS
										RP	N	N	0	NS

(Table 5.3 contd)

Country	Mean age (years)	Years since menopause	Number in group		Study design		Calcium intake (mg/d) (mean)		Duration of supple-mentation (years)	Bone site	Bone loss		Effect of suppl on bone loss	Statistical significance
			Suppl	Unsuppl	R	P	Diet	Supplement			Suppl	Unsuppl		
USA Smith et al 1989 [115]	53	7	44	38	✓	✓	680	1500	4	RP Humerus	Y Y	Y Y	+ +	<0.05 <0.01
Sweden Hansson et al 1987 [116]	66(VF)	nr	22	19	✓	✓	nm	1000	3	LS	N	N	0	NS
Australia Polley et al 1987 [117]	57	8(<10)	34	56	✓	✗	700	1000	0.8	FP	N	Y	+	<0.001
UK Horsman et al 1977 [118]	50	6	24	18	✗	✗	nm	800	2	UD RD MC	Y Y Y	Y Y Y	+ (+) (+)	<0.05 NS NS
USA Recker et al 1977 [119]	57	9	22	20	✓	✗	550	1040	2	RD MC	Y Y	Y Y	0 +	NS <0.05
Australia Nordin et al 1980 [120]	65	20	20	41	✗	✗	nm	1200	variable	MC	(Y)	Y	(+)	NS
Sweden Lamke et al 1978 [121]	60	nr	19	17	✓	✓	nm	1000	1	FN FS	N N	Y Y	(+) (+)	NS NS

Notes: R = randomised; P = placebo controlled; ✓ = yes; X = no; VF = history of vertebral fracture;
NVF = no history of vertebral fracture; nr = not reported; nm = not measured;
NS = no statistically significant difference

Bone loss:
Y = loss significantly different from 0: P<0.05; (Y) = loss >1% per year but NS at P >0.05;
N = significant bone gain, or no bone loss
NS = no statistically significant difference P>0.05

Bone site:
RP = radius proximal; LS = lumbar spine; FN = femoral neck (hip); Troc = trochanter (hip);
Int = intertrochanteric region (hip); W = Ward's triangle (hip); WB = whole body; FP = forearm proximal;
UD = ulna distal; MC = metacarpals; RD = radius distal; FS = femoral shaft

Effect of supplementation on bone loss:
+ = reduced bone loss P <0.05; (+) or (-) = magnitude of difference in loss >1% per year but P > 0.05;
0 = magnitude of diffence in loss <1% per year, P >0.05.
* 1 woman in supplemented group developed milk hypercalcaemia and 44 in supplemented group
(7 in placebo) had hypercalciuria (>35 mg/d)

Table 5.4 Calcium supplementation in women more than 5 years beyond the menopause: controlled studies of the effect on fracture

Country	Mean age (years)	Number in group		Study design		Calcium intake (mg/d) (mean)		Duration of supple-mentation (years)	Fracture site	How fracture diagnosed	% particpants with new fracture		Statistical significance
		Suppl	Unsuppl	R	P	Diet	Supplement				Suppl	Unsuppl	
USA Recker et al 1996 [111]	75 (VF)	53	41	✓	✓	450 (<1000)	1200	4.3	Vertebra	Morphometry	28	51	0.02
	72	42	61	✓	✓	410 (<1000)	1200	4.3	Vertebra	Morphometry	29	21	NS
USA Riggs et al 1998 [114]	66	88	89	✓	✓	710	1600	4*	Vertebra Others	Morphometry Clinical	9 13	10 13	NS NS
New Zealand Reid et al 1995 [108]	58	38	40	✓	✓	700	1000	4	All	Clinical	5	18	0.04
Switzerland Chevalley et al 1994 [112]	72	54	25	✓	✓	620	800	1.5	Vertebra Vertebra Others	Vertebral height Ratio of vertebral heights Clinical	11 20 4	16 44 8	NS <0.05 NS

Notes: R = randomised; P = placebo controlled; ✓ = yes; VF = history of vertebral fracture;
NS = no statistically significant difference
* 1 woman in supplemented group developed milk hypercalcaemia and 44 in supplemented group (7 in placebo) had hypercalciuria (> 35mg/d)

(iii)   The few trials which have used fracture as an end-point have shown small effects from calcium in reducing fracture risk. Again, some of these trials have been performed in healthy women, while others have been performed in those with prevalent vertebral fracture, and all had small sample sizes (see Table 5.4).

5.4.11   *Men*   Twenty five per cent of fractures in people aged 65 years or over are in men. The importance of this public health problem has been overshadowed by the higher rates of fracture in women of the same age. Limited evidence from cross-sectional studies[131,132] confirms that men's bones are affected by a decline in the efficiency of maintaining bone health associated with age, as well as with non-nutritional factors such as smoking and body composition. A study in USA of men aged 30-87 years[133] with a high dietary calcium intake (mean 1159mg/d) found 1 per cent per year bone mineral loss from the radius and 2.3 per cent per year from the vertebrae. The same study could demonstrate no effect in a controlled trial of a combined calcium and vitamin D supplement on bone loss over 3 years (Table 5.5). As with women, bone health may be adversely affected by other diseases and/or therapeutic interventions such as corticosteroids. Men who are hypogonadal have more rapid loss of calcium and bone which can be treated with replacement of testosterone[2].

5.4.12   *Intervention trials with calcium and vitamin D combined (men and women)*   In assessing the influence of specific nutrients on bone health, it is important to avoid confusing the results of trials which are supplemented with single nutrients with those of multi-nutrients. However, for purposes of developing a public health policy, the outcome of trials of supplements which combine the nutrients calcium and vitamin D should also be assessed.

5.4.12.1 *Effects on bone loss*   There have been studies of the effect on bone loss of supplementation with calcium and vitamin D combined using doses of between 500-1200mg calcium taken daily with vitamin D in doses which exceeded the UK RNI (Table 5.5). Bone loss showed no consistent pattern over periods of up to 3 years. In women in USA, whole body bone loss was less in the supplemented group but there were no differences at the femoral neck or the lumbar spine. The results of trials on men are also not persuasive that there is an effect; although the duration of the studies, 3 years, may not be long enough to demonstrate an effect (para 5.4.11).

5.4.12.2 *Effects on fracture incidence*   There have been two longitudinal controlled trials of the effect on fracture of supplementation with vitamin D and calcium combined. The larger in Lyon, France, studied 1765 women aged 69-106 years resident in apartment houses for elderly people or nursing homes. The treated group received 20 µg vitamin D and 1.2g calcium daily. After 18 months, there was significantly lower rate of fracture of hip and of all non-vertebral fractures combined in the supplemented group[133]. Similar results were found after the same study had continued for 3 years[43] (see Table 5.6). The cumulative fracture rates showed divergence of the supplemented and placebo groups at around 8 months for hip fracture and by 3 months for other non-vertebral

Table 5.5 Calcium and vitamin D combined supplementation in older men and women: controlled studies of the magnitude of the effect on bone loss (results presented here have been reworked from the original data)

Country	Mean age (years) and sex	Years since menopause	Number in group		Study design		Dietary calcium intake (mg/d) (mean)	Supplement doses (per day)	Duration of supplementation (years)	Bone site	Bone loss		Effect of suppl on bone loss	Statistical significance
			Suppl	Unsuppl	R	P					Suppl	Unsuppl		
USA Dawson-Hughes et al 1997 [44]	72 (women)	nr	101	112	✓	✓	740	500mg Ca + 17.5µg D3	3	FN LS WB	N N N	N N Y	0 0* +	NS NS <0.001
	71 (men)	-	86	90	✓	✓	710	500mg Ca + 17.5µg D3	3	FN LS WB	N N N	Y N Y	+ + +	<0.001 0.03 <0.001
France Chapuy et al 1992 [133]	84 (women)	nr	27	29	✓	✓	510	1200mg Ca + 20µg D3	1.5	FN Troc Int Total hip	N N N N	N N N Y	+ 0 0 +	0.036 0.044 NS <0.001
USA Orwoll et al 1990 [134]	58 (men)	-	41	36	✓	✓	1160	1000mg Ca + 25µg D3	3	LS RP RD	Y Y Y	Y Y Y	0 0 0	NS NS NS
Australia Nordin et al 1980 [120]	65 (women) VF	20	23	41	X	X	nm	1200mg Ca + 2.5mg-12.5mg vit D	variable	MC	Y	Y	0	NS

Notes: R = randomised; P = placebo controlled; ✓ = yes; X = neither R nor P apply;
nr = not reported; nm = not measured; NS = no statistically significant difference;
VF = history of vertebral fracture

Bone site:
FN = femoral neck (hip); LS= lumbar spine; WB = whole body; Troc = trochanter (hip);
Int = intertrochanteric region (hip); RP = radius proximal; RD = radius distal; MC = metacarpals

Bone loss:
Y = loss significantly different from 0; N = significant bone gain, or loss not significantly different from 0
Effect of supplementation on bone loss:
+ = reduced bone loss; 0 = magnitude of difference in loss <1% per year, $P > 0.05$,
* = significant, positive effect noted after 12 months but not after 3 years

Table 5.6 Calcium and vitamin D combined supplementation in older people: controlled studies of the effect on fracture

Country	Mean age (years)	Number in group and sex		Study design		Calcium intake (mg/d) (mean)		Vitamin D supplementation (per day)	Duration of supplementation (years)	Fracture site	% participants with new fracture		Statistical significance
		Suppl	Unsuppl	R	P	Diet	Supplement				Suppl	Unsuppl	
USA Dawson-Hughes et al 1997 [44]	71	187 (86M+101F)	202 (90M+112F)	✓	✓	710 (M) 740 (F)	500	17.5µg D3	3	Non-vert	5.9†	12.9†	0.02
France* Chapuy et al 1992 [133]	84	877	888	✓	✓	510 (F)	1200	20µg D3	1.5	Hip Non-vert	2.4 7.5	4.2 10.9	0.043 0.015
France* Chapuy et al 1994 [43]	84	872	893	✓	✓	510 (F)	1200	20µg D3	3	Hip Non-vert	12.5 25.0	17.4 31.8	< 0.01 < 0.01

Notes: R = randomised; P = placebo controlled; ✓ = yes; M = Male; F = Female
Non-vert = all non-vertebral fractures (including hip)
† Fractures were more common among the women

fractures. This rapid response suggests that the effect may have been due to an improvement in the myopathy which characterizes vitamin D deficiency. Although the two groups had been shown to be similar at baseline in the proportion who had recent falls, no data were presented on the fall rates in the groups during the study. The most recent study from Boston, USA, recruited healthy volunteers aged 65 years or older[44]. At 3 years the cumulative incidence of non-vertebral fractures in the supplemented group was significantly lower than that in the placebo group. The divergence between the rates of fracture in the supplemented and in the unsupplemented groups was manifest at 6 months. There was no difference in the fall rate between supplemented and unsupplemented groups so this did not account for the observed differences in fracture rates.

In conclusion:

The RNI for calcium for adults, except lactating women, is 700mg/d. Although there has been much debate about whether it represents an adequate intake, the data on which to base proposals for an increase are few. In particular, studies with long term follow-up which use clinical outcome measures are needed. There is evidence that calcium intakes below the current LRNI of 400mg/d might not be compatible with good bone health. The Subgroup therefore did not propose changes to the current DRVs for calcium (conclusion 5.1.3).

5.4.13   *Pregnant women*
           RNI 700mg/d(17.5mmol); LRNI 400mg/d(10.0mmol)

During pregnancy there are major changes in hormonal patterns and metabolism. Maternal plasma calcium concentrations fall by about 5 per cent, a change which is established by 10 weeks gestation and maintained to term. It is thought to follow haemodilution and a reduced protein bound calcium fraction. Active transport mechanisms in the placenta ensure that the fetal plasma calcium levels are maintained at a higher level than maternal, although there is bi-directional flux. Parathyroid hormone (PTH) and calcitonin levels for mother and fetus are independently controlled and neither cross the placenta. The active transport of calcium possibly explains why fetal plasma PTH is lower and calcitonin levels higher than those of the mother. The placenta is capable of synthesising $1,25(OH)_2$vitamin D, and despite a rise in its binding protein, free levels of plasma $1,25(OH)_2$vitamin D increase by up to 70 per cent in normal women during pregnancy. These changes account for the observed increase in efficiency of absorption of calcium from the diet which allows the mother to meet the increased calcium requirements of pregnancy by adaptation without the need for a dietary increment. This occurs without, in most cases, significant reductions in BMD[135] although there are exceptions[74]. A decrease in bone mineral does not necessarily imply that calcium supply is insufficient, nor that increasing the dietary calcium intake will prevent it.

In conclusion:
The factors taken into account by the DRV Panel in 1991 in deciding that the

RNI for calcium during pregnancy should be the same as for adults who are not pregnant were reviewed and confirmed. The Subgroup found no basis on which to recommend otherwise (conclusion 5.1.4).

5.4.14   *Lactating women*
                                RNI 700mg/d(17.5mmol); plus increment 500mg/d(14.3mmol)

There is no evidence that lactation, even when frequent and prolonged, has a long term influence on the bone health in later life of individual women. Lactation is commonly but not invariably associated with bone mineral changes during the first 3 to 6 months which are related to the volume of breast milk produced[135]. The reduction in bone mineral, where this occurs, may amount on average to 4 per cent in the spine but is much less on a whole body basis[136]. The decrease in bone mineral is observed in populations with low and high calcium intakes and is not affected by calcium supplementation[137] (Table 5.7). The decrease is reversed towards the end of lactation and after cessation of breastfeeding[138]. For women who become pregnant during or shortly after lactation there is evidence that the recovery of bone mineral occurs during the subsequent pregnancy[139]. These data, which have become available since the UK DRVs were last reviewed, suggest that additional calcium intake during lactation is not required for long term bone health. No decision was made to remove the increment during lactation pending the outcome of other long term studies now in progress.

In conclusion:

The UK RNI for calcium during lactation includes an additional 550mg/d derived factorially. Recent data suggest that this increment might not be necessary. The Subgroup considered it prudent to await further data before deciding whether to revise this increment (conclusion 5.1.5).

Table 5.7 Longitudinal studies during lactation to assess relationship between calcium intake and bone changes

Country	Number in group			Post partum age at start of study	Calcium intake (mg/d) at 1-3 month lactation (mean)	Bone site	Correlation between bone change and calcium intake
	Breastfeeding	Mother not breastfeeding	Not recently pregnant or lactating				
Observational studies							
England Laskey et al 1998 [137]	47	11	22	2 week	1250	LS, hip, WB, RS, RD	0
USA Krebbs et al 1997 [143]	26	8	-	0.5 week	1390	LS, RS	0$
Chile Lopez et al 1996 [140]	30	-	26	4 week	1480	LS, hip	0
USA Sowers et al 1993 [142]	90	20	-	2 week	1320	LS, hip	0
USA Hayslip et al 1989 [141]	12	7	-	2 day	1790	LS, RS, RD	0
**Supplementation studies ** **							
USA Kalkwarf et al 1997 [76]	87 / 76	81 / 82	- / -	2 week / 4-6 month	740 (+1000***) / 690 (+1000***)†	RS, RD, LS, WB / RS, RD, LS, WB	0* / 0*
Australia Kent et al 1995 [144]	79	-	-	1 week	1050 (+1000***)	LS, hip, FD, FS	0
The Gambia Prentice et al 1995 [145]	60	-	-	1.5week	280 (+700***)	RS, RD	0
USA Cross et al 1995 [146]	15	-	-	<2 week	1300 (+1000***)	LS, WB, RS, RD, US, UD	0

Notes: All studies demonstrated significant changes in bone mineral at one or more skeletal site in lactating women that were not seen in the controls.

Bone site:
LS = lumbar spine; WB = whole body; RS = radius shaft; RD = radius distal; FD = forearm distal;
FS = forearm (radius + ulna) shaft; US = ulna shaft; UD = ulna distal

Correlation:
0 = none; + = smaller decrease in bone mineral associated with higher calcium intake.
* Ca supplementation increased bone mineral density at the lumbar spine in both lactating and non-lactating women, but had no effect on the patterns of change post-partum.
** Randomised placebo controlled. *** Intake during study. † In supplemented group.
$ Significant association of BMD and calcium intake in the lactating women but not on the bone change.

6. Reassessment of the DRVs for vitamin D

6.1 Conclusions

6.1.1   The RNI for vitamin D of 10 μg/d continues to be recommended for pregnant and lactating women (para 6.4.2).

6.1.2   The RNI for vitamin D for the first 3 years of life continues to be appropriate without change in the levels. It is acknowledged that the majority can maintain an adequate vitamin D status without supplementation, but a substantial minority remains vulnerable (para 6.4.3).

6.1.3   There has been no new evidence to suggest that individuals aged 4-64 years rely on dietary intake for adequate vitamin D status, which is generally achieved through the action of sunlight. However, specific groups including women who wear clothes intended to conceal themselves fully, especially if they have had pregnancies unsupplemented with vitamin D may be at risk.   Consequently, there was no evidence on which to base a recommendation to change the zero RNI for vitamin D (with 10 μg/d for those at risk).   The DRVs for the population aged 4-64 years should remain unchanged (para 6.4.6).

6.1.4   The RNI for people aged 65 years or over of 10 μg a day should be retained.   It reflects a prudent public health approach to safeguard against vitamin D deficiency and its adverse effect on bone health.   No data have been presented to suggest a change in the level.   For a majority of people in this group vitamin D supplementation will be needed to achieve this intake (para 6.4.10).

6.2   Metabolism of vitamin D and bone status

6.2.1   There are two forms of vitamin D.   Cholecalciferol (vitamin D_3) is synthesised through the action of light of wavelengths between 290nm and 310nm on 7-dehydrocholesterol in the skin of animals, including humans. Ergocalciferol (vitamin D_2) is synthesised in plants and fungi by irradiation of plant steroid ergosterol.   In humans synthesis in the skin provides the major contribution of vitamin D, but the smaller dietary component is also very important.   Neither vitamins D_3 or D_2 have biological effect until they are converted to 25 hydroxychole(or ergo)calciferol (25(OH)vitamin D_3 or D_2) in the liver, and then to 1,25dihydroxychole(or ergo)calciferol (1,25(OH)$_2$vitamin D_3 or D_2) in the kidney[147].   The rate of conversion to 1,25(OH)$_2$vitamin D by the kidney is PTH dependent (para 3.3.4).

6.2.2   The active hormonal form, 1,25(OH)$_2$vitamin D, controls plasma calcium concentrations by modulating calcium absorption in the small intestine, phosphate resorption in the renal tubules and through calcium release from bone. A specific nuclear receptor for 1,25(OH)$_2$vitamin D (vitamin D receptor) occurs in tissues involved in calcium homeostasis, such as intestine, kidney and bone. 1,25(OH)$_2$vitamin D also appears to promote calcium deposition in growing ends of bones but the mechanisms are not fully understood but may be mediated via an effect on osteocalcin concentrations[148]. 1,25(OH)$_2$vitamin D has several other functions not specifically related to calcium; deficiency causes impaired function of nerves and muscles, as well as behavioural changes such as depression. A specific nuclear vitamin D receptor has been identified in a variety of non-calcaemic tissues including placenta, gonads, skin and cells of the immune system.

6.2.3   *25(OH)vitamin D as an indicator of vitamin D status*   Plasma levels of the active form of vitamin D (1,25(OH)$_2$vitamin D) are under homeostatic control, which limits their value as a marker of status. Consequently the conventional marker of vitamin D status is plasma 25(OH)vitamin D. This intermediary is responsive to changes in dietary vitamin D and to exposure to sunlight. Plasma levels of 25(OH)vitamin D found in clinical rickets or osteomalacia range from undetectable to around 20nmol/l[17] and a level of plasma 25(OH)vitamin D of 25nmol/l has conventionally been used as a cut off for defining the lower limit of adequacy of vitamin D status[25], although others have suggested slightly higher levels[149]. There are no data relating plasma levels of vitamin D above those associated with clinical disease to long term bone health.

6.2.4   Recent data relating plasma levels of PTH to those of 25(OH)vitamin D have led to the suggestion that elevation of PTH might define the level of 25(OH)vitamin D needed for bone health, beyond the avoidance of clinical deficiency[150]. It has long been the prevailing opinion that the plasma level of calcium is the major determinant of plasma PTH levels and an oral calcium load can reduce PTH[151]. However, more recent data suggest that plasma PTH levels may rise in response to poor vitamin D status. Studies show a consistent inverse association between plasma levels of 25(OH)vitamin D and of PTH in a variety of different age and sex groups. In addition, supplementation with 10 µg vitamin D can reduce plasma PTH levels[152]. However, use of the plasma level of PTH as a marker of vitamin D status is hindered by a number of uncertainties.

6.2.5   Firstly, it is unclear whether there is an "optimal" level of plasma 25(OH)vitamin D above which plasma PTH remains at a lower plateau level and below which PTH rises. A number of studies report an inverse association between plasma 25(OH)vitamin D and serum PTH without identifying a threshold[151,152,153,154,155,156,157]. One small short term intervention trial reported a reduction in plasma PTH after oral vitamin D and calcium only in people whose pre-treatment plasma 25(OH)vitamin D was below 50nmol/l[158]. Where a threshold for plasma 25(OH)vitamin D has been identified, this varies between studies from less than 20nmol/l to 110nmol/l[147,159,160,161,162].

6.2.6   Secondly, there is large variation in the plasma levels of 25(OH)vitamin D which is associated with any particular level of PTH[157,162]. This variation lowers the confidence which can be placed in deriving a cut off. The large variation is confirmed by the low correlations reported between plasma levels of PTH and of 25(OH)vitamin D, usually of the order of r = -0.2[152,153,156] though both stronger[151], and weaker correlation coefficients[155], have been reported. Theoretical calculations based on this observed relationship have led to the suggestion that "normalising" plasma PTH would require intakes of vitamin D in excess of those currently recommended in the US (10 μg/day)[157], while others report that the seasonal variation of plasma PTH is abolished in those with habitual vitamin D intakes of 5 μg/day[163].

6.2.7   Finally, there is insufficient evidence to identify levels of plasma PTH (below those characteristic of clinical hyperparathyroidism) which may have adverse effects on bone health, nor on the time needed for any such effect to occur. While it has been proposed that, at least in women, higher levels of plasma PTH, lower levels of plasma 25(OH)vitamin D and seasonal variations in them, on the one hand, lead to bone loss, lower bone mineral density and/or fracture, on the other[161], there are insufficient data to establish with certainty a particular level of plasma PTH which carries adverse effects, and which could currently be used to define vitamin D insufficiency.

6.2.8   In conclusion, there are now considerable data indicating that plasma levels of PTH rise with poor vitamin D status. However, a number of other factors, including dietary calcium intake, also affect plasma PTH. In addition, because of considerable uncertainty in the data, it is not yet possible to define a threshold level of plasma 25(OH)vitamin D at which PTH begins to rise. Finally, the possibility that levels of plasma PTH below those found in clinical hyperparathyroidism, but above those found in healthy young people, might lead to adverse effects, remains uncertain. Consequently, the Subgroup felt unable to use the plasma PTH data to define a lower cut off for adequacy of plasma 25(OH)vitamin D, and agreed to use the conventional level of 25nmol/l in their assessment of the vitamin D status of the UK population.

6.2.9   *Influences of season and latitude*   Due to its northerly latitude (between 50°N and 60°N), ultraviolet light of appropriate wavelength is only at sufficient intensity in Britain, between beginning April and mid October (Fig 6.1). Seasonal variations in blood 25(OH)vitamin D levels were first identified in 1974[164,165] which confirmed that sunlight is a major factor in determining vitamin D status. Unless the diet is supplemented, vitamin D requirements during winter must be provided from the vitamin store accumulated during the previous summer's exposure. It has been estimated that to maintain plasma levels of 25(OH)vitamin D above 20nmol/l (8 μg/l) during winter, levels during summer must be greater than 40nmol/l (16 μg/l)[166].

6.2.10   The degree of seasonal variation in plasma 25(OH)vitamin D level can be used to assess the effects of latitude on the rate of skin synthesis of vitamin D. European, Scandinavian and North American populations all reflect a significant

Figure 6.1 Mean effective ultraviolet radiation (UVR) irradiance* at 3 UK sites

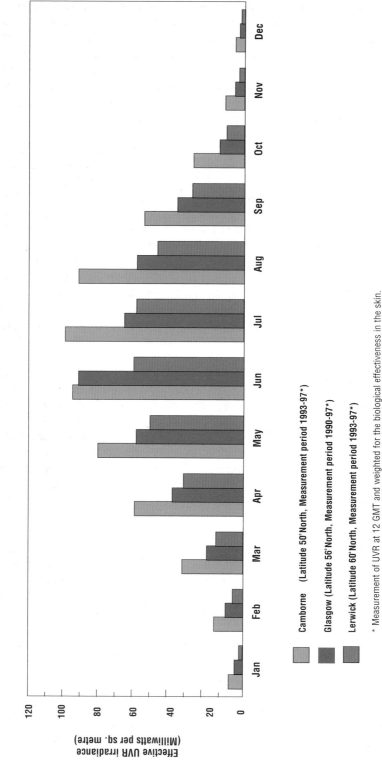

Camborne   (Latitude 50°North, Measurement period 1993-97*)

Glasgow (Latitude 56°North, Measurement period 1990-97*)

Lerwick (Latitude 60°North, Measurement period 1993-97*)

* Measurement of UVR at 12 GMT and weighted for the biological effectiveness in the skin.
Source: National Radiological Protection Board (unpublished data)

seasonal variation in vitamin D status. In several countries nearer to the equator, such as Mexico and Saudi Arabia (both latitude 20°S), the vitamin D status of the population also reflects the season of the year. In others there is no evidence of seasonal variation, for example in Brazil (latitude 8°S) children had similar mean values of 25(OH)vitamin D in winter and summer and these were at least twice as high as the vitamin D levels in British children[167]. In the Gambia (latitude 13°N) the 25(OH)vitamin D concentrations of women were similar across the seasons and matched those of British women during the summer[168].

6.2.11   The seasonal effect on vitamin D status implies an increased risk of inadequate status during the winter months in latitudes distant from the equator. The fall in serum 25(OH)vitamin D levels and increase in PTH levels in winter[163] has been prevented by dietary supplementation with vitamin D at levels of 10 µg per day[169]. A randomised controlled trial in 189 healthy British men and women aged 63-76 years showed that a single oral dose of 2.5mg (100,000 IU) of vitamin D_3 raised serum 25(OH)vitamin D levels by 60 per cent and reduced serum PTH levels by 12 per cent in five weeks[32]. An older group of people living in institutions in Rochdale, UK, maintained satisfactory plasma concentrations of 25(OH)vitamin D throughout the year on a twice yearly oral dose of 2.5mg vitamin D. A dose given once a year appeared to be inadequate for this group who were never exposed to sunlight, because 40 per cent had low plasma levels for a period of the year[170].

6.2.12   There was a seasonal variation in hip fracture rate in Newcastle but whether this relates to seasonal variations in vitamin D status is not known[171]. It appeared to comprise two separate effects: one cluster of hip fractures in December and January with falls out of doors, possibly associated with social and shopping activities at Christmas, and a second cluster of fractures incurred by falls indoors, in early spring, possibly attributable to falls resulting from neuromuscular changes of vitamin D deficiency. On the other hand, in North America the magnitude of the seasonal variation in hip fracture incidence was unchanged over a range of latitudes and showed no association with presumed levels of sunlight exposure[172].

6.2.13   *Variations in vitamin D metabolism associated with age*   As the skin ages it is less efficient at synthesising vitamin D under the influence of sunlight[172] because the thickness of the epidermis declines with age and the amount of the vitamin D precursor 7-dehydrocholesterol is reduced[174].   Gastrointestinal absorption of vitamin D is also less efficient in older people[175] and age-associated reductions in 1 alphahydroxylase in the kidney may impair the conversion of 25(OH)vitamin D to $1,25(OH)_2$vitamin D[176]. There is also an age-associated decline in the trophic effect of PTH in enhancing the production of $1,25(OH)_2$vitamin D in the kidney[176].

6.2.14   *Variations in vitamin D metabolism associated with skin pigmentation*
The amount of melanin in the skin influences the capacity to synthesis vitamin D. Synthesizing equivalent quantities of cholecalciferol requires longer exposure to ultraviolet light if the skin is more pigmented. However, the eventual blood

concentrations of 25(OH)vitamin D following unlimited exposure are the same in all races[177]. This means that certain ethnic minority groups in the UK are more vulnerable to vitamin D deficiency than is the majority white group[159,178]. As well as a more pigmented skin, there are several cultural features distinctive to these populations which also influence vitamin D status adversely including wearing clothes which conceal[179], a tradition of not spending time out of doors, and dietary differences, particularly excluding meat and fish from the diet[178,180].

6.2.15   *Adverse effects of high vitamin D intakes*   Vitamin D is toxic in large doses. Hypervitaminosis D is characterised by high serum levels of 25-hydroxyvitamin D and hypercalcaemia or hypercalciuria, or both. Prolonged hypervitaminosis D can result in calcium deposition in the soft tissues, changes in the central nervous system, and, in severe cases, death. In most individuals there has to be very high levels of vitamin D intake before there are signs of hypervitaminosis D but there are cases of infantile hypercalcaemia being caused by moderate increase in vitamin D intakes[11]. In America, between 1987 and 1991, a home delivery dairy accidentally overfortified cows' milk with vitamin D. The level of vitamin D in the samples of milk tested was 70 to 600 times higher than the 10µg per quart recommended for fortification (approximately 635 to 7400µg/l).   Of the 56 cases of hypervitaminosis D in the delivery area of the dairy diagnosed between 1985 and 1991, 19 of the patients were customers of the dairy, hypervitaminosis D occurred most frequently in patients taking prescribed vitamin D supplements and 62 per cent of the patients were older than 60 years[181]. A review of studies of the effectiveness and safety of continuous low-dose (20-45µg) and intermittent high-dose (2.5-15mg) vitamin D supplementation in elderly people reported 3 cases of hypercalcaemia out of 442 patients. Two cases were associated with a predisposing cause and an underlying cause, the third was not investigated[182].

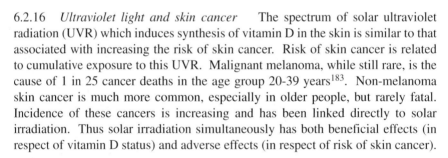

6.2.16   *Ultraviolet light and skin cancer*   The spectrum of solar ultraviolet radiation (UVR) which induces synthesis of vitamin D in the skin is similar to that associated with increasing the risk of skin cancer. Risk of skin cancer is related to cumulative exposure to this UVR. Malignant melanoma, while still rare, is the cause of 1 in 25 cancer deaths in the age group 20-39 years[183]. Non-melanoma skin cancer is much more common, especially in older people, but rarely fatal. Incidence of these cancers is increasing and has been linked directly to solar irradiation. Thus solar irradiation simultaneously has both beneficial effects (in respect of vitamin D status) and adverse effects (in respect of risk of skin cancer).

6.2.17   The UK Skin Cancer Prevention Working Party has prepared a Consensus Statement about the importance of measures to reduce exposure to UVR. It stresses the greater risk to the skin of children under 15 years and dispels any misconception that a tanned skin is either a sign of health or that it provides more than minimal protection against further exposure.

It puts forward a four point plan to moderate sun induced skin damage:

- avoid noonday sun (between 11.00 am and 3.00 pm),

- seek natural shade,

- use clothing as a sunscreen,

- use a broad spectrum sunscreen of high sun protection factor.

In developing local policies it is important to strike a balance between these constraints, which are aimed at reducing the risk of skin cancer, and the need to ensure an adequate vitamin D status from exposing some skin to sunlight regularly during the months of May to September[184]. The Subgroup recommends that the public health consequences of sunlight exposure should be reviewed to take account of both its beneficial and its adverse effects with a view to developing guidelines. The effect on vitamin D status of measures taken to reduce the risk of skin cancer, such as encouraging covering up with clothes and applying cosmetic creams which seek to prevent the UVR reaching the skin should be clarified.

6.3   Dietary Reference Values for vitamin D: a review of the evidence

6.3.1   Plasma 25(OH)vitamin D is a good marker of vitamin D status but the assay has only recently become widely available and there are several population groups with no data for this marker.   The relationships between plasma 25(OH)vitamin D, 1,25(OH)$_2$vitamin D and PTH are beginning to be explored. The DRVs for vitamin D set in 1991 were determined on the basis of that dietary amount required to ensure that plasma 25(OH)vitamin D levels in winter did not fall below 20nmol/l (8 μg/l)[17].

6.3.2   In reviewing the DRVs for vitamin D, two questions are relevant. Is an RNI needed? If so, is the current value correct? In assessing the need for vitamin D in regard to bone health, particular search was made for reports of longitudinal and intervention trials. In some trials the vitamin D supplement amounted to no more than the UK RNI and there were few data from trials using supplements which exceeded the current RNI.

6.4   Dietary Reference Values for vitamin D for different population groups

6.4.1   *Pregnant and lactating women*
RNI 10 μg/d

A mother provides a store of vitamin D to her fetus during pregnancy. In order to meet this demand, pregnant women should be well provided with vitamin D themselves. The majority of pregnant women appear to have no difficulty in maintaining their own vitamin D status satisfactorily, as well as providing for their fetus, but a substantial minority are vulnerable to deficiency because of the season of the year, latitude of abode, skin pigmentation[14,21,185] and dietary[185] and other cultural habits[31].

6.4.2   The arguments in support of setting an RNI for women who have recently given birth are not very secure. A dietary source of vitamin D will ensure that women, vitamin D depleted as a result of pregnancy, are restored to an adequate status. Good vitamin D status of the mother during lactation might be expected to influence the infant's vitamin D status, but little vitamin D is available from breast milk. Maternal vitamin D status and dietary vitamin D intake both influence breast milk concentrations of 25(OH)vitamin D but there is no correlation between the levels in breast milk and plasma 25(OH)vitamin D status of breastfed infants except when the mother consumes high dose vitamin D supplements[186]. An RNI of 10 µg/d for all pregnant and recently delivered women represents a prudent approach[187]. In practice this means that vitamin D supplements are advised[188].

In conclusion:

The RNI for vitamin D of 10 µg/d continues to be recommended for pregnant and lactating women (conclusion 6.1.1).

6.4.3   *Children aged 0-3 years*
            0-6 months: RNI 8.5 µg/d
            6 months-3 years: RNI 7 µg/d

It is important that children under 3 years maintain satisfactory vitamin D status to meet the demands of rapid growth. From about age 6 months if infants are out of doors some of the time and especially if it is summer or are consuming vitamin D rich weaning foods in good amounts they should be adequately provided for. However, exposure to sunlight must be moderated because at this age children are very vulnerable to skin damage and sunburn (para 6.2.16). Several groups of infants and younger children are at risk of vitamin D deficiency for a variety of reasons. This is increased if the mother's vitamin D status in pregnancy has been inadequate to provide the fetus with a store sufficient to last during the early months of life, if it is winter and if the infant's diet contains no meat or vitamin D rich foods[188]. The risk is not limited to the ethnic minority groups. In the absence of vitamin supplementation more than one factor may operate to render an individual child particularly at risk of deficiency[189].   Routine vitamin D supplementation, as recommended in the Department of Health report Weaning and the Weaning Diet[188] will achieve the RNI, and forms an effective safety net for groups at risk.

In conclusion:

The RNI for vitamin D for the first 3 years of life continues to be appropriate without change in the levels. It is acknowledged that the majority can maintain an adequate vitamin D status without supplementation, but a substantial minority remains vulnerable (conclusion 6.1.2).

6.4.4   *Older children*
            No RNI is set for older children

The current DRV recommendations are that there is no need for a dietary source of vitamin D to maintain an adequate vitamin D status in this age group except for specified at risk groups. There is no new evidence to change this recommendation.

6.4.5 Adults aged 18-64 years
No RNI is set

No RNI is set for adults aged 18 to 64 years. The majority of this adult population can obtain an adequate vitamin D status if the skin of the face and arms is exposed for about half an hour a day between April and October. It is important to avoid sunburn which may occur with this exposure in late spring and high summer (para 6.2.17). There are no representative data about the vitamin D status of this group of adults in this country. There is no evidence to suggest that the younger members of this group might be vitamin D deficient provided vulnerable groups (para 6.4.6) are considered separately. However, between ages 45 to 65 years vitamin D status may start to decline, possibly associated with lifestyle changes including not going outdoors and not exposing skin to the same extent as at younger ages. Further data are needed, especially on plasma 25(OH)vitamin D levels, before it would be possible to consider whether this older group might need a dietary source of vitamin D and at what intake level.

6.4.6   People who hardly ever go outdoors will be vulnerable as will those who wear clothes to conceal themselves fully when they are outside[190]. More information is needed about the vitamin D status of vulnerable groups in the population. There are no data from representative surveys either about dietary practices, supplement taking or plasma 25(OH)vitamin D levels. For some women who already have a vitamin D status which is borderline for sufficiency, one or more pregnancies, especially if not supplemented, may result in frank deficiency of vitamin D and osteomalacia. In all these circumstances, vitamin D supplements are recommended for these vulnerable but minority groups.

In conclusion:

There has been no new evidence to suggest that individuals aged 4-64 years rely on dietary intake for adequate vitamin D status, rather it is achieved through the action of sunlight, except for specific at risk groups including women who wear clothes intended to conceal themselves fully, especially if they have had pregnancies unsupplemented with vitamin D. Consequently, there was no evidence on which to base a recommendation to change the zero RNI for vitamin D (with 10 µg/d for those at risk). The DRVs for the population aged 4-64 years should remain unchanged (conclusion 6.1.3).

6.4.7 Older adults
From age 65 years RNI 10 µg/d

For people of 65 years or older, the RNI for vitamin D is 10 µg/d. Older people engage in less physical activity and go out of doors less than younger groups[191] and there is reduced efficiency of vitamin D synthesis in the skin (para 6.2.13). A study of older people in nursing or other institutional homes compared a daily dose of 10 µg with a daily dose of 20 µg vitamin D. It was concluded that the 10 µg dose was sufficient to lower the parathyroid hormone levels and to improve vitamin D status as measured by increases in plasma 1,25(OH)$_2$vitamin D levels especially in those who had been deficient before the start of the study[152]. The Subgroup found no new evidence on which to base proposals for a change in the RNI.

6.4.8   Several studies have found that mean plasma levels of 25(OH)vitamin D are lower in patients with hip fracture than in women without fracture[192]. This may reflect a causal relationship or may be due to the higher fracture rates of old people who are relatively immobile and housebound. Studies from the north of England in the 1970s found that a proportion, 20 to 47 per cent, depending on criteria, of elderly people with hip fracture had histological evidence of osteomalacia[193]. More recent studies have found lower prevalences, 2 per cent in Cardiff[194] and 12 per cent in Leeds[195]. Clinical observations in Tyneside (UK) (EH Jarvis personal communication) suggest that the incidence of frank osteomalacia has fallen in the last twenty years among the elderly population despite the rise in incidence rates of proximal femoral fracture in this group[171]. Thus it is likely that frank osteomalacia makes only a minor contribution to the total risk of hip fracture. On the other hand, it is probable that the long term adverse effect of repeated winters characterised by several months of deficient vitamin D status, secondary hyperparathyroidism and loss of bone, contributes to the development of osteoporosis[155,196].

6.4.9   Vitamin D supplementation trials

6.4.9.1 *Vitamin D supplementation trials and bone loss*   Rickets and osteomalacia are cured by vitamin D therapy but these conditions are rare. Three trials have evaluated the effect of vitamin supplements on age related bone loss as assessed by bone scans. Only one trial in very elderly women, gave vitamin D alone and that at the level of the UK RNI[160] (Table 6.1). The results suggested that the supplemented group had significantly less bone loss at the femoral neck. The remaining two trials[169,197], both in younger women, showed no effect of vitamin D supplements given for two years on bone loss. In each trial additional calcium was given to both groups whether supplemented with vitamin D or not.

6.4.9.2 *Vitamin D supplementation trials and fracture*   There has been one randomised placebo controlled clinical trial of vitamin D supplementation and fracture incidence. This study in Amsterdam recruited a group of people over 70 years who were reasonably active in their own homes or in institutions; half took 10 µg vitamin D supplement a day, the rest took a placebo. After 36 months, there was no difference in the fracture rate between the supplemented and the unsupplemented groups[198]. An earlier study in Finland recruited very elderly people, some living in their own homes and some in institutions[199]. Vitamin D was given to half the group as an intramuscular injection once a year and the unsupplemented group received nothing.   After 40 months, there was a significantly higher rate of fractures, taking all sites together, in the unsupplemented group.   The differences between the supplemented and unsupplemented groups for hip fracture did not achieve statistical significance, although there was a significantly higher rate of fractures of the upper limbs (Table 6.2). The cumulative incidence rates of fracture in treated and untreated groups began to diverge at 6 months in the group of people living in institutions, and at 18 months in the group living in their own home. This would appear to indicate too rapid an effect to be mediated by change in BMD and raises the possibility that part of the benefit arose from reducing fall rates as vitamin D supplementation improved neuromuscular coordination. This more immediate effect of vitamin D supplementation in those in institutions may have been related to their presumed greater degree of vitamin D deficiency.

6.4.10   *Intervention trials with vitamin D and calcium combined*   These have been described at para 5.4.12 and also Tables 5.5, 5.6. There have been two trials which showed a reduction of fracture rate over 3 years in the supplemented groups with vitamin D doses at or close to 20 µg daily and calcium supplements of 1.2g in one study[43,133] and 0.5g[44] in the other. Other trials of combined vitamin D and calcium showed no consistent effect on the magnitude of bone loss.

In conclusion:

The RNI for people aged 65 years or over of 10 µg a day should be retained. It reflects a prudent public health approach to safeguard against vitamin D deficiency and its adverse effect on bone health. No data have been presented to suggest a change in the level. For a majority of people in this group vitamin D supplementation will be needed to achieve this intake (conclusion 6.1.4).

Table 6.1 Vitamin D supplementation in postmenopausal women: controlled studies of the magnitude of the effect on bone loss (results presented here have been reworked from the original data)

Country	Mean age (years)	Years since menopause	Number in group		Study design		Calcium intake (mg/d) (mean)	Vit D suppl μg/d	Duration of supple-mentation (years)	Bone site	Bone loss		Effect of suppl on bone loss	Statistical significance
			Suppl	Unsuppl	R	P					Suppl	Unsuppl		
Netherlands Ooms et al 1995 [160]	80	32	177	171	✓	✓	870**	10D3	2	FN Troc RD	N (Y) N	(Y) (Y) Y	+$ 0 +	0.001 NS NS
USA Dawson-Hughes et al 1991 [169]	64	15	(a) 123 (b) 124	- -	✓	X	460+ 500*	(a) 17.5 D3 (b) 2.5 D3	2	LS FN WB	(a) (b) N N Y Y N N		0 +† 0	NS 0.003# NS
Denmark Christiansen et al 1980 [197]	45-54	0.5-3	28	121	✓	✓	diet+ 500*	50 D3	2	FD	Y	Y	0	NS

Notes: R = randomised; P = placebo controlled; ✓ = yes; X =neither R nor P apply;
NS = no statistically significant difference: D3 = cholecalciferol

Bone site
FN = femoral neck (hip); Troc = trochanter (hip); RD = radius distal; LS = lumbar spine;
WB = whole body; FD = forearm distal

Bone loss
Y = loss significantly different from 0; (Y) = loss >1% per year but NS; N = significant bone gain,
or loss not different from 0

Effect of supplementation on bone loss:
+ = reduced bone loss ; 0 = magnitude of difference in loss <1% per year, P >0.05
* Both the vitamim D supplemented and the placebo groups recived additional calcium as supplements.
** = calcium intake from dairy products
$ = Supplement effect was greater in the first year.
† = positive effect of the higher dose compared to the lower dose.
# = effect was greater in year 1

50

Table 6.2 Vitamin D supplementation of old people: controlled studies of the effect on fracture

Country	Mean age (years)	Number in group		Study design		Calcium intake (mg/d) (mean)	Vitamin D suppl	Duration of supplementation (years)	Fracture site	% participants with new fracture		Statistical significance
		Suppl	Unsuppl	R	P					Suppl	Unsuppl	
Netherlands Lips et al 1996 [198]	80 (M+F)	834	792	✓	✓	870	10µg/d D3	3	Hip Non-vert	7.0 16.2	6.1 15.4	NS NS
Finland Heikinheimo et al 1992 [199]	86 (M+F)	341	458	✓	X	nm	3.75-7.5mg once a year* D2	3.3	Upper Limbs Hip All	2.9 7.3 16.4	6.1 9.4 21.8	0.025 NS 0.034

Notes: M = male; F = female; R = randomised ; P = placebo controlled; ✓ = yes;
X = neither R nor P apply; nm = not measured; Non-vert = all non vertebral fractures
including hip
NS = no statistically significant difference P>0.05.
* = given by annual intramuscular injection

51

7.   Other influences on bone health

7.1   Genetic influences

7.1.1   Genetic influences make an important contribution to the variations in bone status between healthy individuals. Broadly speaking, African-Caribbean racial groups tend to have larger and heavier bones than White or Asian populations, and there is also diversity within populations and between men and women. Family studies have made some progress in clarifying the polygenic inheritance of bone size and strength[200]. Mutations of collagen regulating genes have been associated with inherited pathological disorders known as osteogenesis imperfecta which give rise to severe osteoporosis[201]. Recently, evidence from a case-control study suggested that other mutations of the same gene might be associated with reduced bone density and/or fracture in the vertebrae of otherwise healthy women[202].

7.1.2   Other candidate genes extend across the spectrum of metabolic events concerned with the maintenance of bone integrity. The oestrogen receptor gene is polymorphic. In a Japanese population, lower BMD was associated with a particular oestrogen receptor gene polymorphism[203]. Polymorphisms of the vitamin D receptor (VDR) gene have been correlated with BMD in some studies and may be useful in predicting fracture risk[204] however other studies have failed to confirm this association[205]. The racial, dietary and other environmental differences between the populations being studied may have influenced the correlations between the VDR polymorphism and BMD[206]. For example, calcium intake may interact with the effect of the VDR genotype on BMD so that postmenopausal bone status only correlates where there is a low calcium intake[207,208] and the low calcium intakes may need to have been prolonged. Variation in calcium intake is but one of many likely confounding factors.

7.2   Nutritional influences other than calcium and vitamin D

7.2.1   *Body composition*   BMC and BMD are influenced by overall body size and weight. Higher lean-to-fat ratio protects bone in younger women and in men, whilst the reverse is true for older women[209,210]. Tall stature is a risk factor for hip fracture[6], whilst small, thin women are at greater risk of vertebral fracture. Thus lean body mass and body size, in addition to adiposity, are also important factors in bone health. Anorexia nervosa is associated with a lower than expected bone mass and an increased risk of fractures[211]. There is a lack of prospective data in this area, but it is reasonable to conclude that it is undesirable for older people to be underweight.

7.2.2   *Nutrients other than calcium and vitamin D*   Nutrients other than calcium and vitamin D are undoubtedly important in determining bone health[212]. The Subgroup was not able to assess their influence in detail. The data about individual nutrients are sparse, usually observational rather than from intervention trials, and based on small numbers. There are no long term data from controlled trials. In spite of these limitations, it has been possible to make a brief comment about the nutrients that have been linked to bone health at least through preliminary findings.

7.2.2.1 *Protein*   There is inconsistent evidence about the relationship between protein intakes and bone health. Elderly patients with hip fracture are often undernourished at admission to hospital; those given protein-rich nutritional supplements showed improved clinical outcome[213]. Some studies in women have associated higher intakes of protein with increased fracture risk[214,215] and lower BMD[216], while others suggest the reverse[94] or no association[217].

7.2.2.2 *Vitamin K*   Vitamin K status might influence bone health as several vitamin K-dependent proteins, including osteocalcin and matrix gla-protein, are involved in bone mineralisation[218,219]. Low dietary intake of vitamin K is associated with an elevated proportion of under-carboxylated (partially functional) osteocalcin[220] and this has been associated with low BMD and increased risk of hip fracture[221,222,223] in older women.

7.2.2.3 *Vitamin C*   Vitamin C is required for collagen hydroxylation. There are limited human studies on vitamin C and bone health: cross-sectional studies report positive associations with a trend to higher BMD with increased vitamin C intake in adolescents[224] and middle-aged premenopausal women[225], but no association in postmenopausal women[226].

7.2.2.4 *Magnesium, phosphorus*   There has been only limited study of relationships between bone status and minerals other than calcium. Magnesium is widely distributed in soft and bony tissue. Low serum magnesium levels have been reported in women with osteoporosis[227], and there may be a positive association between magnesium intake and BMD in middle-aged premenopausal women[225]. Phosphorus as phosphate makes up roughly half the weight of bone. The evidence on whether phosphorus intake has any effect on bone health is inconsistent[94,216,217].

7.2.2.5 *Sodium, potassium*   Increasing dietary sodium intake results in increased urinary calcium excretion, and a direct relationship is found between urinary excretion of sodium and of calcium in free-living populations[228]. This effect may be particularly pronounced in some individuals[229]. It has been suggested that this might influence BMD[230,231] but the evidence is not conclusive[232]. There is some evidence that in middle-aged women higher dietary potassium intake has been associated with higher BMD[225,233]. These observations suggest that current recommendations for healthy eating[234,235] which advise a reduction in the average intake of sodium from about 150mmol/day to 100mmol/day and an increase in average intakes of potassium to about 90mmol/day would have no detrimental effect on bone health and might be beneficial.

7.2.2.6 *Fluorine*   Fluoride incorporation into bone results in atypical alignment of the apatite crystals[236,237]. A recent American consensus statement concluded that the levels of fluoride likely to be obtained from fluoridated water supplies are unlikely to influence bone health[238]. Population studies in different countries report both positive and negative effects of fluoride on BMD and fracture risk, with no accord on the effective level of fluoride[239]. Recent low dose trials (25-50mg sodium fluoride daily) appear to suggest reduced fracture incidence[240]. The first study to consider the role of fluoride intake from all sources (foods, water and non-dietary) on hip fracture is ongoing. On current information, estimated maximal intakes in the UK[17] appear to be below the level likely to influence bone health.

7.2.2.7 *Other nutrients*   Other nutrients which might have a plausible biochemical basis for influencing bone health include zinc[241,242], copper[243], B vitamins[244,245], manganese[227] and boron[246]. There is only very limited information relating to possible independent effects on bone health of these nutrients. Zinc is known to affect infant growth which could be through indirect mechanisms such as appetite or through direct effects on bone[80]; a positive association has been noted between higher intakes of zinc and BMD in middle-aged premenopausal women[247]. In the genetic condition, Menkes' syndrome, copper deficiency causes characteristic bone defects that can be detected by x-ray[248]. A controlled trial of copper supplementation in middle aged women showed no loss in BMD in the copper supplemented group compared to a significant decrease in BMD in the placebo group[243]. A positive effect on spinal bone density was found with the combination of calcium, zinc, manganese and copper in a small trial in healthy postmenopausal women[249]. There is currently insufficient evidence to support dietary recommendations in relation to the effect of any of these nutrients on bone health.

7.2.3   *Vegetarian diets*   Interpretation of the effects of a vegetarian diet on bone health is difficult because of other differences, such as body weight, socio-economic status, physical activity and smoking habits, that may be associated with a vegetarian lifestyle. There is no evidence that a lactovegetarian diet is associated with differences in bone mineral density or fracture risk[250,251]. There is little information about those eating a vegan or macrobiotic diet, but two recent studies have reported lower bone densities in adolescents and older women in association with these diets[210,252].

7.3   **Other dietary components**

7.3.1   *Alcohol*   Heavy alcohol consumption is associated with decreased BMD and modestly increased fracture risk[253]. The influence of moderate alcohol consumption is unclear and has been associated with both higher BMD[225] and lower BMD[94,254].

7.3.2   *Caffeine*   The effect of caffeine on bone health is difficult to assess as high caffeine intake is often associated with other risk factors. Oral doses of caffeine increase the urinary excretion of calcium[228]. High caffeine has been associated with decreased BMD in postmenopausal women who have low calcium intakes[255,256]. In pre- and perimenopausal middle aged women a negative association between caffeine intake and BMD was found[217]. A study of postmenopausal women found no association between caffeine intake and BMD[257].

54

7.3.3 *Phytoestrogens* Phytoestrogens are widely distributed plant chemicals which can cause oestrogenic effects. Phytoestrogens are capable of binding to the oestrogen receptor but in many tests *in vivo* and *in vitro* are considerably less physiologically potent than endogenous oestrogens. However, comparatively large amounts are found in foods, and there are differential binding effects in the alpha and beta oestrogen receptor[258]. Animal studies report that the phytoestrogen genistein is as active as oestrogens in maintaining bone mass in ovariectomised rats[259]. Data in humans are too limited to draw conclusions.

7.4 Hormonal and reproductive factors

7.4.1 During childhood there is a continual process of bone growth and modelling which is influenced by growth and thyroid hormones, $1,25(OH)_2$vitamin D and other hormones. There are spurts of bone growth in the preschool years and at puberty. Bone growth may slow during a period of illness followed by accelerated growth on recovery. This is probably mediated by hormonal influences and it is likely that the associated physical inactivity and use of medicines are also causes of these changes.

7.4.2 Both male and female hormones exert anabolic effects on bone, and for both men and women, a decline in the level of sex hormones is associated with bone loss[260]. Thus, women at the menopause, and men who become hypogonadal both experience bone loss which is hormone dependent and separate from the bone loss which is age related. Bone loss, particularly trabecular, accelerates in the years following the menopause[261] and there is increased bone turnover with an increase in the rate of formation of both osteoclasts and osteoblasts[262]. These changes can be modified by therapeutic oestrogen replacement[1].

7.5 Smoking

7.5.1 Smoking has been suggested as a possible factor which increases the risk of osteoporosis[263]. The studies are limited to observational data of different types (cohort, case control and cross-sectional) and so are liable to confounding by various aspects of lifestyle and health associated with smoking, in particular poorer micronutrient status and body weight. Smokers tend to be lighter, which is independently a risk factor for fracture (para 7.2.1). There is some evidence that an effect of smoking on bone health might be mediated via oestrogen antagonism[264,265]. A recent meta-analysis of data from 48 such studies relating smoking to BMD in long bones and to hip fracture[266] found that smoking had little independent effect on BMD or hip fracture in women before the menopause. Other data confirm that an apparent effect of smoking in premenopausal women is abolished after correction for body weight[267]. However the meta-analysis confirmed an effect of smoking on BMD and hip fracture in postmenopausal women, and from more limited data, in men, independent of thinness, age of menopause, physical activity or oestrogen status. Other data suggest a similar or greater effect on fracture at vertebral and radial sites[268]. Smoking does not appear to influence peak bone mass, but may have a direct effect on the rate of bone loss in older age.

7.6   Physical activity

7.6.1   There is long standing recognition, particularly from epidemiological observations, that physical activity protects against risk of fracture in postmenopausal women[268,269]. Since physical activity is a lifestyle factor which can be modified, it is important to identify the nature and level of those activities which may influence risk. It is also important to determine the duration of participation in the physical activities before a beneficial effect occurs and whether such benefit persists beyond cessation of the activities.

7.6.2   The loading on the bone either from gravitational forces, or from muscular tension influences its functional strength[270]. Both arise through weight bearing activities such as running, climbing stairs and jumping, while weight-training (lifting weights) involves muscular tension alone. Most activities have both weight bearing and non-weight bearing components, for instance, racket sports. In general, weight bearing activities have a positive effect in increasing BMD in young women[271] and premenopausal women[272] and in helping to maintain BMD after the menopause[273]. Dynamic exercises which increase the loading on the weight bearing skeleton show a maximum effect from high impact activities such as jogging and jumping[273,274,275,276]. Walking, though weight bearing, needs to be brisk to have an effect on BMD[277]. Muscular activities without weight bearing or impact, such as swimming[278] and cycling[279] do not influence BMD. Weight-training is sometimes found to increase or maintain BMD[280,281] although many good studies show no effect despite large gains in muscle strength[282,283]. If the activities are discontinued in favour of a sedentary lifestyle, any improvements in bone or muscle are gradually lost[275].

7.6.3   An active lifestyle at all ages promotes good general health, and diverse physical activities bring benefit to the health not only of bones, but also of other body systems. All physical activity contributes to energy expenditure (which is desirable), and moderate activity, whether weight bearing or not, promotes cardiovascular health. Physical activity such as walking may stimulate appetite. This would be valuable for those elderly people whose low food intakes makes nutrient inadequacies more likely. Walking at a normal pace appears not to confer benefit for BMD except perhaps in those who are extremely sedentary (i.e. walking less than 10 minutes per day in total), but it does contribute to improved balance and muscle coordination, which in turn might help to prevent the falls which precipitate fractures.

7.6.4   Participation for about 30 minutes in varied physical activities with a weight bearing component on five days a week would be expected to promote stronger bones. Examples include:

• *for children and young adults*: high impact activities such as jogging, jumping or skipping and games which require these such as basketball, also energetic dancing;

- *for middle-aged people*: stair climbing, jogging, or walking briskly, ideally on a gradient, step exercises, racket sports and hill walking;

- *for older people*: stair climbing and walking as briskly as is realistic and safe, also dancing.

Particular precautions are needed to ensure that the activities are of an intensity appropriate for the age and capability of the individual. A brisk walk implies a pace of at least four miles per hour[284] which is not advisable if it leads to an increase in the fall rate. High-impact weight bearing activity would be precluded for those with established osteoporosis or arthritis. However, more moderate supervised activities benefit the person's confidence and mobility and may lead to fewer fractures[2].

8. Assessment of nutrient intakes and nutritional status of the population

8.1   **Monitoring food and nutrient intakes** (see Annex 3)

8.1.1   The British National Food Survey (NFS) began in 1940 and since 1996 also covers Northern Ireland. It is a continuous survey of all food entering the home for human consumption for seven days and records the description, quantity and cost. Nutrient intakes assessed from the NFS do not include nutrients derived from dietary supplement use. Some 8000 households in Britain take part every year. From 1992 it has also recorded food purchased and consumed outside the home. The survey is particularly helpful in assessing time trends in food consumption and nutrient intakes but it does not provide information about the food and nutrient intakes of individuals[285].

8.1.2   Diet and nutrition surveys of large numbers of individuals are complex and expensive. The most recent nationally representative data for Britain were obtained on adults aged 16-64 years in 1986/7[286], children aged 1½-4½ years in 1992/3[287] and people aged 65 years or over in 1994/5[288]. Fieldwork for a comparable survey of young people aged 4-18 years was completed in early 1998. Data on trends in food and nutrient intakes, or nutritional status, are less easy to derive from these infrequent surveys. Some comparative data are beginning to be built up and the results of the survey of preschool children in 1992/3[287] can be compared with those from a survey of children of similar ages in 1967/8[289]; also the results of the survey of older people in 1994/5[288] can be compared with a survey in 1972/3[290]. The National Diet and Nutrition Surveys (NDNS) are designed to provide nutrient intake data both from diet and from supplements for each age group that are representative of the population. As fieldwork is spread over 12 months, seasonal variations can also be examined. More details about the surveys are given in Annex 3.

8.1.3   Surveys need to be sufficiently large and representative of their target group to provide information of value for public health purposes. The sample sizes for the NDNS are insufficient to provide reliable data on population subgroups such as those from an ethnic minority, disabled people, people on diets which regularly exclude food items for cultural, religious or medical reasons, or other small groups in the population. Several local surveys have examined the food and nutrient intakes of individuals from such smaller specific population subgroups.

8.1.4   There are occasions where apparent discrepancies arise between the results of the NFS and NDNS. These are generally due to differences in the design and structure of the surveys, and may also arise due to changes in dietary habits since the earlier surveys were conducted.

8.1.5   Only data from the UK have been included in the analyses tabulated in this report. In spite of increasing international flows of food and cuisine, national public health policies for nutrition must be based on current national diet and nutrition data. This does not, however, imply that inter-country comparisons are invalid for assessing the scientific basis of the recommendations.

8.1.6   *The composition of foods*   Reliable and up-to-date information on the nutrient content of foods is essential to estimate nutrient intake from food consumption data collected in dietary surveys. In the UK, there is an ongoing programme to monitor the nutritional value of the foods that make up the national diet. This programme is continuous as the range and type of foods available, their composition, and their relative importance in the diet are continually changing. In addition, methods of food analysis are improving all the time. The data collected from this analytical programme and other sources (e.g. from food manufacturers) are used to compile nutrient databanks for both the NFS and the NDNS. In addition, the information is incorporated into the UK food composition tables, McCance and Widdowson's "The Composition of Foods" series. Recent changes in vitamin D content of meat illustrate the importance of continuously updating information on the nutritional value of foods. Measurable amounts of vitamin D and its metabolites have now been found in carcase meat as a result of new analytical methods. The use of these new data on vitamin D in meat in the National Food Survey resulted in a considerable increase in assessed vitamin D intake in 1995 (Table 10.1).

8.1.7   *Dietary supplements*   In the UK dietary supplements are classed as foods, and are subject to the general provisions of the Food Safety Act 1990. Products with a significant pharmacological effect or where medicinal claims are made (e.g. implicit or explicit claims that the product is capable of treating, curing or preventing human disease) would be subject to controls under medicines legislation. They would require Product Licences under the Medicines for Human Use (Marketing Authorisations etc.) Regulations 1994 to be licensed for certain clinical indications and may be prescribed by doctors to individuals for specific uses.

8.2   Assessing the adequacy of a population's diet

8.2.1   Good data about the customary diet and nutritional status of a population are prerequisites for the development of national public health policies for nutrition. The DRVs provide benchmark levels of nutrient intakes against which to compare mean values for population intakes. Policies for population subgroups, such as older women or adolescents, require specific information about that group's current dietary habits and nutritional status. It is important that the data are as up-to-date as possible and based on a sufficiently large and representative sample of the population group. The British NDNS programme seeks to adhere to these principles. In practice the dietary data from populations do not always meet these ideals. The information may have been based on very small numbers of participants, or they may not have been representative of their sector of the population. The data may not be up-to-date and, as a result, may not reflect dietary habits of today.

8.2.2   Misreporting of food consumption can occur in dietary surveys. Participants may forget or otherwise omit to record some items consumed and so underreport their intake. Overreporting can also occur if, for example, food left on the plate is not taken into account. In such circumstances confidence might be reduced in the accuracy of a group mean level of intake for a nutrient. One approach to explore whether there has been underreporting is to compare, retrospectively, an individual's recorded energy intake with their basal metabolic rate (BMR) calculated from their weight using Schofield's equations[17] and weight and height for older people[184]. If an apparently healthy individual has recorded a diet which provided an energy intake no more than 1.2 times their calculated BMR (representing a minimum ratio of energy intake to BMR compatible with ordinary life over prolonged periods), the record may not reflect habitual dietary intake. A decision can then be made whether to exclude these individuals from comparison with the DRVs or alternatively their energy and nutrient intakes may be adjusted. The value 1.2 times BMR is an arbitrary choice and similar calculations can be applied using a more conservative value of 1.4 times BMR to judge the quality of a dietary record. Manipulating data from a survey by excluding individuals brings the likelihood of introducing new errors. In general, applying maximum effort to collecting an accurate dietary record is preferable, and this is the approach of the NDNS.

8.2.3   *Markers to assess nutritional status*   As well as assessing nutrient intakes as a reflection of likely nutritional status, a range of physiological markers has been developed to assess nutritional status by examining body fluids such as blood and urine. New assays are more widely available. For example, measures of iron status from blood analysis have been used for a long time, but plasma 25(OH)vitamin D assays are more recent although the significance of the results obtained from the newer assays continue to be evaluated (para 6.2.3), the new status markers are already contributing to more accurate assessments of nutritional status. These measures complement traditional clinical methods for diagnosing gross nutritional disorders such as rickets, anaemia due to iron or vitamin B_{12} deficiency, or obesity. There are no recognised markers of calcium status (para 9.2.1).

9. Dietary intake and nutritional status of the population - calcium

9.1   **Conclusions**

9.1.1   There are no functional tests for adequacy for calcium status; therefore this can only be assessed as intake against reference values (para **9.2.1**).

9.1.2   The calcium intakes of infants and children up to age 4½ years are adequate as assessed against the DRVs (para **9.10.2**).

9.1.3   There are no recent data about calcium intakes in primary school children. Data about older children are limited to specific ages and, because they were collected several years ago, may not reflect current dietary practices. It is not possible to draw firm conclusions for this age group but average intake was below RNI values in secondary school children, especially older girls, and all young people should take special care to avoid low calcium intakes. When the data from the National Diet and Nutrition Survey of young people are available, they should be reviewed with particular reference to calcium intakes and to identifying the characteristics of those whose intakes are low (para **9.10.3**).

9.1.4   The calcium intakes of adult women are adequate compared to DRVs, although intakes of a proportion of women particularly in the younger groups are low. However, underreporting may account for some of the apparent low intakes. A National Diet and Nutrition Survey of adults aged 19-64 years is now being planned to begin fieldwork in 1999 and should provide more up-to-date data from which calcium intake can be assessed. Meanwhile, it is prudent for those with low calcium diets to increase their intake (para **9.10.5**).

9.1.5   A proportion (less than 10 per cent) of older women in Britain not living in institutions appear to have calcium intake levels which are low as assessed against DRVs (para **9.10.6**).

9.1.6   There is no evidence that the diets of pregnant or lactating women do not provide adequate intakes of calcium (para **9.10.7**).

9.1.7   In general, the calcium intakes for men appear to be adequate at all ages although there was a small proportion with intake below the LRNI (para **9.10.8**).

9.2   **Assessing calcium status**

9.2.1   There is no biochemical indicator of calcium nutritional status. The plasma calcium level is highly conserved and urinary calcium levels are influenced by many factors. As a result the calcium status of population groups can only be assessed from the total calcium intake from diet and supplements.

There are no adequate functional tests for adequacy for calcium status; therefore this can only be assessed as intake against reference values (conclusion 9.1.1).

9.3   **Calcium intakes of the British population**

9.3.1   *Calcium intake from household foods*[285]   The current average household calcium intake in the population is around 820mg/day (Table 9.1). The major dietary sources of calcium in British household diets are milk and milk products (approx 56 per cent) and cereals (approx 25 per cent, with about 14 per cent from bread due to calcium fortification of "white" flour). There has been a decline in total calcium intakes since 1975 of around 200mg/day which corresponds with the decline in total milk and bread consumption. Over the same period there were no changes in the calcium density of the diet as energy intakes have also declined (Fig 9.1).

9.3.2   *Calcium in water*   Calcium from drinking water is well absorbed[291]. The contribution of water to nutrient intake is generally not assessed in dietary surveys. The calcium content of water varies from region to region; very hard

Figure 9.1 Calcium content of British household food (1975-1996)

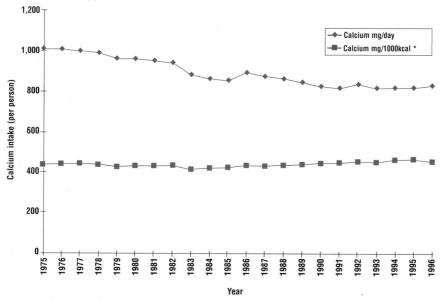

* calcium density of the diet
Source: MAFF, National Food Survey 1975-1996 (see para 8.1.1)

Table 9.1 Contributions made by selected foods to the calcium content of food purchased by British households - 1970-96 (averages)

Food Source	Year													
	1970		1975		1980		1985		1990		1995		1996	
	mg/d	%	mg/d	%	mg/d	%	mg/d	%	mg/d	%	mg/d	%	mg/d	%
Total milk & milk products	618	59.0	623	61.7	572	59.9	479	56.5	473	57.9	470	58.3	462	56.3
- liquid whole milk	464	44.3	476	47.2	416	43.5	285	33.6	207	25.3	137	17.0	131	16.0
- skimmed & semi skim	-	-	-	-	-	-	41	4.8	125	15.3	195	24.2	190	23.2
- cheese	112	10.7	112	11.1	117	12.2	116	13.7	102	12.5	94	11.7	96	11.7
Total Cereals	259	24.7	227	22.5	222	23.2	216	25.5	201	24.6	191	23.7	207	24.7
- "white" bread	138	13.2	115	11.4	84	8.8	79	9.3	61	7.5	59	7.3	49	6.0
- other bread	21	2.0	22	2.2	29	3.0	45	5.3	54	6.6	51	6.3	64	7.8
- cakes, pastries, biscuits	40	3.8	40	4.0	38	4.0	34	4.0	33	4.0	33	4.1	37	4.5
- flour	37	3.5	32	3.1	54	5.7	40	4.7	29	3.5	19	2.3	22	2.7
- breakfast cereals	n/a	n/a	n/a		n/a		5	0.6	8	1.0	6	0.7	10	1.2
- other cereals	22	2.1	20	2.0	16	1.7	13	1.5	16	1.9	23	2.8	26	3.1
Vegetables	62	5.9	57	5.6	61	6.4	53	6.3	50	6.1	47	5.8	50	6.1
Meat, fish & products	38	3.6	37	3.7	41	4.3	40	4.7	37	4.5	42	5.2	44	5.4
Eggs	20	1.9	16	1.6	14	1.5	13	1.5	9	1.1	8	1.0	8	1.0
Fruit & fruit products	19	1.8	16	1.6	17	1.8	15	1.8	17	2.1	18	2.2	18	2.2
Total beverages	8	0.8	7	0.7	8	0.8	7	0.8	7	0.9	7	0.9	7	0.9
Other	23	2.2	26	2.6	21	2.2	24	2.8	23	2.8	23	2.9	24	2.9
Total daily calcium intakes (mg)	1047		1009		956		847		817		806*		820*	

Notes: Figures may not add up due to rounding. No data on skimmed milks are available before 1985 but skimmed milks were available in small quantities in the early 1980s with consumption increasing during the decade. n/a = data not available. * Since 1992 nutrients obtained from soft and alcoholic drinks and confectionery, and food and drink consumed outside the home have also been assessed. These are excluded from the table but accounted for an extra 88mg of calcium a day in 1995 and 74mg in 1996
Source: MAFF: National Food Survey, 1970-1996 (see para 8.1.1)

63

water from the Cotswolds can contain around 300mg calcium per litre and soft water in Lancashire may contain virtually no calcium. The water consumed as tap water, in dilutable soft drinks and coffee or tea is likely to be locally drawn, but the water in ready-to-drink soft drinks, beer and bottled water may come from a remote source where it was manufactured and/or bottled. In addition the water used in the manufacture of soft drinks and beer might be treated to remove ions, for example de-ionised or treated by reverse osmosis. This makes it difficult to assess the calcium intake from water and water-based drinks. The total liquid (including water) consumed by an adult is around 1.5-2litre/day. In a survey of South Northumberland adolescents it was calculated that they obtained 8 per cent of their dietary intake of calcium from non-milk beverages due to a local water supply containing 300mg of calcium per litre[292].

9.4   **Calcium intakes in specific population groups** (Table 9.2)

9.4.1   *Infants*   Average calcium intakes in 1986 were 744mg per day for infants aged 6-9 months and 825mg calcium per day for those aged 9-12 months[293].

9.4.2   *Preschool children*   For preschool children aged 1½-4½ years the mean calcium intake in 1992/3 was 637mg/day. The main sources were milk and milk products providing an overall average of 64 per cent of the calcium intake (contributing 70 per cent at 1½-2½ years, 63 per cent at 2½-3½ years and 59 per cent at 3½-4½ years) and cereals, which provided an overall average of 19 per cent of the intake (contributing 16 per cent at 1½-2½ years, 20 per cent at 2½-3½ years and 23 per cent at 3½ -4½ years). The mean intakes decreased with age, particularly when variations in energy intake and body weight were taken into account[287]. Mean calcium intakes for preschool children were about 5 per cent lower in 1992/3 than in 1967/8[289].

9.4.3   *School children*   In 1983, mean daily calcium intakes for boys were 833mg at age 10-11 years and 925mg at 14-15 years. For girls the mean values were lower, 702mg at 10-11 years of age and 692mg at 14-15 years of age[294].

9.4.4   *Young adults*   A survey in 1982 of young British adults reported mean daily intakes of 1000mg and 885mg for males and females respectively aged 15-18 years. Values for age 19-21 years were similar at 1100mg and 745mg, and for 22-25 years were 1125mg and 880mg for males and females respectively[295].

9.4.5   *Adults*   In 1986/7, in a national Dietary and Nutritional Survey of British Adults (aged 16-64 years), the average intake of calcium from food sources only (i.e. excluding dietary supplements) was 937mg/day for men and 726mg/day for women[286].

9.4.6   *Older adults*   In 1994/5, the NDNS of people aged 65 years and over[288] found a mean daily intake of calcium from food sources in those not living in residential or nursing institutions (free-living) of 852mg in 65-74 year old men, 813mg in 75-84 year old men and 764mg in men over 85 years. There was a similar age related decline in women's daily intakes from a mean of 704mg to 680mg to 647mg in respective age groups. Both men and women who lived in institutions had higher mean intakes of calcium than their free-living age related peers, in excess of 800mg/day. Calcium intakes of older people not living in institutions were lower in 1994/5 than in 1972/3[290]. Participants not living in

Table 9.2 Mean daily calcium intakes (mg) in Britain by age and sex

Age Group	Year of fieldwork	Sex	Number in group	Mean calcium intake mg/d	
				Total from food sources (1sd)	from supplements
6 - 9 months [293]	1986	Male	130	760 (236)	n/a
		Female	128	729 (254)	n/a
9 - 12 months [293]	1986	Male	96	849 (269)	n/a
		Female	134	808 (271)	n/a
6 - 18 months [289]	1967/8	Male	103	771* (n/a)	-
		Female	96		
1½ - 2½ years [289]	1967/8	Male	186	691* (n/a)	-
		Female	181		
2½ - 3½ years [289]	1967/8	Male	188	658* (n/a)	-
		Female	194		
3½ - 4½ years [289]	1967/8	Male	164	661* (n/a)	-
		Female	142		
1½ - 2½ years [287]	1992/93	Male	298	682 (278)	1
		Female	243	643 (266)	0
2½ - 3½ years [287]	1992/93	Male	300	642 (251)	1
		Female	306	628 (268)	0
3½ - 4½ years [287]	1992/93	Male	250	625 (226)	0
		Female	243	595 (212)	0
10 - 11 years [294]	1983	Male	902	833 (253)	-
		Female	821	702 (217)	
14 - 15 years [294]	1983	Male	513	925 (303)	-
		Female	461	692 (223)	
15 - 18 years [295]	1982	Male	197	1000 (n/a)	n/a
		Female	184	885 (n/a)	
19 - 21 years [295]	1982	Male	104	1100 (n/a)	n/a
		Female	119	745 (n/a)	
16 - 24 years [286]	1986/7	Male	214	894 (337)	5
		Female	189	675 (267)	0
22 - 25 years [295]	1982	Male	149	1125 (n/a)	n/a
		Female	158	880 (n/a)	n/a
25 - 34 years [286]	1986/7	Male	254	931 (318)	2
		Female	253	699 (267)	1
35 - 49 years [286]	1986/7	Male	346	960 (306)	1
		Female	385	760 (270)	4
50 - 64 years [286]	1986/7	Male	273	949 (269)	3
		Female	283	739 (217)	8
65 - 80 years [290] not in institutions	1972/3	Male	111	890 (285)	-
		Female	125	780 (251)	
81+ years [290] not in institutions	1972/3	Male	58	870 (311)	-
		Female	71	690 (184)	
65 - 74 years [288] not in institutions	1994/5	Male	271	852 (285)	1
		Female	256	704 (237)	8
75 - 84 years [288] not in institutions	1994/5	Male	265	813 (290)	0
		Female	217	680 (256)	4
65 - 84 years [288] living in institutions	1994/5	Male	128	935 (338)	1
		Female	91	900 (261)	2
85+ years [288] not in institutions	1994/5	Male	96	764 (252)	0
		Female	170	647 (253)	7
Living in institutions		Male	76	981 (295)	2
		Female	117	828 (271)	7

Note: n\a = data not available, * = data not available for males and females separately
Older reports give mean values for total calcium intakes which include intakes from both food and supplements, but values are not reported separately from these two sources.
sd = standard deviation.

institutions obtained about 50 per cent of their calcium intakes from milk and milk products and about 25 per cent from cereals and cereal products. Those living in institutions obtained a similar proportion from milk and somewhat more from cereals at about 35 per cent of intake for men and 30 per cent for women. Further information about the reported calcium intakes of older people in diverse circumstances is set out in Table 9.3.

Table 9.3 Mean daily calcium intakes (mg) in Britain by age and sex for specified groups of older people

Age Group	Year of fieldwork	Region	Other characteristics	Number studied	Mean calcium intakes (1sd) or [95% confidence limits]
65+ years	1991/2[301]	Edinburgh	*In sheltered housing*		
			males	54	858 (336)
			females	160	731 (300)
68 - 90 years	1990[302]	Norwich	*Not in institutions*		
			males	60	889 [852 - 928]
			females	85	805 [777 - 835]
50 - 85 years	1985-7[188)]	Southampton	*Not in institutions*		
			males	120	843* [560-1042]
			females	480	651* [467 -799]
63 - 89 years	1985[303]	Southampton	*Healthy* (70 - 85 years)	24	1004 (100)
			Housebound (70 - 85 years)	20	800 (132)
			Hospitalised, non-smokers (63 - 89 years)	21	792 [700 -888]
65 - 95 years	1974-6[304]	Belfast	*Institutionalised:*		
			- in hospital		
			males (+Suppl)*	11	970 (246)
			females (+Suppl)*	43	854 (122)
			males	13	791 (88)
			females	30	763 (141)
			- in residential accommodation		
			males	9	892 (82)
			females	17	868 (142)
			- in sheltered dwellings		
			males	3	619 (243)
			females	17	654 (223)
			Residing at home		
			males	10	1000 (398)
			females	27	711 (285)
			males (+Suppl)**	5	668 (154)
			females (+Suppl)**	11	719 (305)

Notes: * = subjects taking multivitamin supplements for at least 3 months prior to study
** = calcium intakes estimated from frequency and amount questionnaire providing information on the consumption of milk, bread, cheese, puddings, cakes and biscuits
sd = standard deviation

9.4.7   *Pregnant women*   Several local dietary studies of pregnant women have shown mean calcium intakes of about 900mg/day in the first trimester, with intakes increasing to 1000mg/day or more as pregnancy advances (Table 9.4) which can be attributed to changes in eating habits, including slight increases in intakes of milk, milk products and bread[296,297,298,299].

9.4.8   *Lactating women*   Calcium intakes at two months postpartum of women in Edinburgh and London were assessed according to whether the participant was lactating or not[296]. Mean daily calcium intakes, which were lower than those reported by the same women during pregnancy (Table 9.4), were higher in lactating women in London (880mg) than in Edinburgh (857mg), likewise in non-lactating women: London, 780mg and Edinburgh, 671mg. In both cities whether lactating or not, mean calcium intakes were lower for women from lower social classes. The study of pregnancy and postpartum calcium intakes from Cambridge reported higher intakes during lactation but confirmed the lower intakes in women from "manual occupation" families: 1500mg/day non-manual, 1400mg/day manual[300]. In a more recent study, also from Cambridge, the mean daily calcium intake for lactating women was 1250mg[77].

Table 9.4 Mean daily calcium intakes (mg) in Britain of pregnant women

Stage of pregnancy	Year of field work	Region	Special characteristics	Number in group	Mean calcium intakes mg/d (1sd)
Early	1987/8[298]	Aberdeen	in early pregnancy attending antenatal clinic	50	860 (295)
1st trimester	1986[296]	London and Edinburgh	living in London living in Edinburgh	46 87	873 (n/a) 964 (n/a)
1st trimester	1980[305]	Hackney and Hampstead London	delivered infant birthweight ≤2500g birthweight 3500-4500g	28 165	761(n/a) 953(n/a)
2nd trimester	1986[296]	London and Edinburgh	living in London living in Edinburgh	91 36	983 (n/a) 911 (n/a)
2nd trimester	1982-4[306]	South London	smokers non-smokers	94 112	910 (330) 1030 (349)
3rd trimester	1991/2[307]	South-west England	longitudinal study of pregnancy and childhood	11,923	953 (500; 1442)*
3rd trimester	1987/8[299]	Aberdeen	attending antenatal clinic	224	1015 (357)
3rd trimester	1986[296]	London and Edinburgh	living in London living in Edinburgh	110 107	1045 (n/a) 988 (n/a)
3rd trimester	1984/5[297]	Aberdeen	married women booked for hospital delivery	142	980 (463)
3rd trimester	1982-4[306]	South London	smokers non-smokers	72 97	840 (314) 990 (304)
stage not stated	1986 [300]	Cambridge	non-manual occupation manual occupation	42 21	1300 (300) 1100 (300)
stage not stated	1977-1980 [308]	Harrow London	attending antenatal clinic all Asian Hindu vegetarians Hindu non-vegetarians Muslim non-vegetarians White	813 450 225 138 54	1186 (410) 1253 (417) 1165 (375) 1002 (389) 1127 (489)

Notes: n/a = data not available; sd = standard deviation; * 5th and 95th percentiles

9.5   Contribution to calcium intakes from fortification

9.5.1   Within the cereals group more calcium is supplied from "white bread" than any other category, due to calcium fortification of "white"[***] flour which also accounts for the high proportion of calcium obtained from buns, cakes, pastries, biscuits, puddings, other bread such as brown and continental types and other cereal products such as pizza. The proportionate contribution to mean calcium intakes from fortified flour was estimated from data collected in three nationally representative diet and nutrition surveys[286,287,288].

Population group	Estimated percentage of calcium intake from fortified flour
1½-2½ years male and female	12%
2½-3½ years male and female	17%
3½-4½ years male and female	19%
16-64 years male	13%
16-64 years female	11%
65+ years male (not in institutions)	13%
65+ years female (not in institutions)	11%
65+ years male (living in institutions)	12%
65+ years female (living in institutions)	11%

9.6   Contribution made by dietary supplements to the total calcium intake

9.6.1   The National Diet and Nutrition Surveys assess the contribution of supplements to nutrient intakes (Table 9.2). In the recent survey of people aged 65 years and over calcium supplements (including prescribed supplements) contributed 2 per cent of total calcium intake for women not living in institutions. When prescribed supplements were excluded the contribution was reduced to 1 per cent of total calcium intake.   For women in institutions supplements contributed 1 per cent of total calcium intake (0.5 per cent when prescribed supplements were excluded). The contribution made by supplements to intakes for men in this age group was negligible. Calcium supplement taking was uncommon at all ages but was most likely in older women and was more common in individuals who were already towards the higher end of the range of calcium intakes. Of those not in institutions 4.3 per cent (48 of 1110 survey participants) of individuals took calcium supplements, as did 2.8 per cent (10 of 357 survey participants) of individuals living in institutions.

9.7   Regional variations in calcium intakes

9.7.1   Mean daily calcium intakes assessed from household foods vary from 790mg in Scotland to 860mg in the East Midlands, but there is no regional trend[285] (Figure 9.2). This generally matches the findings from surveys of individuals (Table 9.5) although there are age related regional differences. Preschool children and adults (including older people) had lower intakes in Scotland and Northern England compared with the intakes in the Midlands, Wales and Southern England. The surveys of school children and young people generally found higher calcium intakes in Scotland and the North.

[***] "White" flour includes all flour except wholemeal and certain specialised flours.

Figure 9.2 Calcium content of British household food by region (1994-1996)

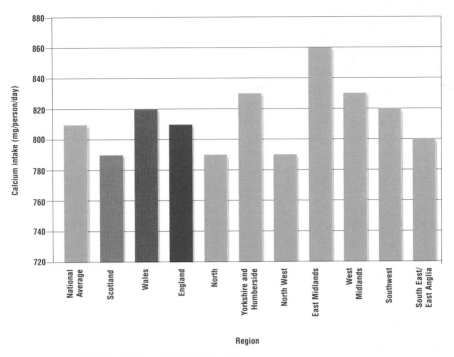

Source: MAFF, National Food Survey 1994-1996 (See Para 8.1.1)

Table 9.5 Mean daily calcium intakes (mg) from all sources (includes supplements) by age, sex and region of Britain

Age Group	Year of field work	Sex	Region			
			Scotland	England and Wales		
				Northern	Central, South-West & Wales	London & South-East
1½ - 4½ years	1992/3[287]	Both	614	629	639	651
10 - 11 years	1983[294]	Male	880	830	810	700
		Female	740	710	690	660
14 - 15 years	1983[294]	Male	960	900	940	920
		Female	720	609	710	660
15 - 25 years	1982[295]	Male	1255	1140	1070	1090
		Female	800	880	830	845
16 - 64 years	1986/7[286]	Male	881	888	968	967
		Female	692	705	750	738
65+ years *not in institutions*	1994/5[288]	Male	777		878	857
		Female	667		695	730

69

9.8 Variations in calcium intakes with social class/income

9.8.1 Surveys of individuals show an association between low calcium intake and lower social class (assessed on occupation of the head of household) although the sizes of the groups for Class V were generally small (Table 9.6). The National Food Survey assesses intakes by income of the head of household. On this basis mean daily calcium intakes in lower income groups appeared to be somewhat higher than in higher income groups but the differences are small (Figure 9.3). Differences in methodology mean the results from the two types of survey are not directly comparable.

Table 9.6 Mean total daily calcium intakes (mg) from all sources (includes supplements) by age, sex and social class of head of household

Age Group	Year of field work	Sex	Social Class					
			I	II	IIINM	IIIM	IV	V
6 - 9 months	1986[293]	Both		721			757	
9 - 12 months	1986[293]	Both		812			831	
1½ - 4½ years	1992/3[287]	Both		656			623	
10 - 11 years	1983[294]	Male	930	910	770	810	820	810
		Female	740	740	740	700	660	680
14 - 15 years	1983[294]	Male	1100	970	1050	930	870	760
		Female	730	750	670	720	660	600
15 - 25 years	1982[295]	Male	1215		1030	1180	1030	
		Female	930		920	820	735	
16 - 64 years	1986/7[286]	Male	1006		912	917	868	
		Female	790		747	702	660	
65+ years not in institutions	1994/5[288]	Male	885			802		
		Female	745			655		

Notes: NM = non manual occupation; M = manual occupation

Figure 9.3 Calcium content of British household food by income group (1994-1996)

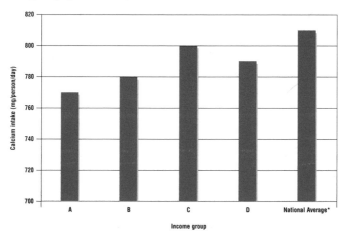

The level of income decreases from income group A to income group D
* National average also includes households without an earner and pensioner households, who had higher calcium intakes than households with an earner.

Source: MAFF, National Food Survey 1994-1996 (See para 8.1.1)

9.9 The diets of minority groups

9.9.1 *Vegetarians*   More than half of the calcium consumed by the British population is from dairy products. Vegetarians who exclude all animal products from their diet (vegans) may have low calcium intakes[310]. In addition, the higher phytate content of a plant based diet may adversely affect calcium bioavailability (para 5.2.3). Average daily calcium intakes of vegans have been reported as 582mg (males) and 497mg (females)[311]. Vegetarians who consumed dairy products had intakes of calcium comparable to those of the general population (Table 9.7).

9.9.2 *Diets from the Indian subcontinent*   The UK population includes minority groups from very many countries. The diets of these groups differ from the diet of the average population to varying extents. There are no representative data about particular ethnic minority diets except that limited information is available for the minority community originating from the North Indian subcontinent ("Asian") (Table 9.7).

9.9.3   Asian infants aged 6 months in Rochdale[312] had lower intakes of calcium than the population average[293], but by 9 months the mean intake was comparable to the national level. During pregnancy Asian women had average intakes of calcium comparable with those of pregnant white women (Tables 9.4 and 9.7).

Table 9.7 Mean daily calcium intakes (mg) of adult vegetarians and of young children and pregnant women from the Indian subcontinent now living in Britain

Population Group	Year of fieldwork	Special characteristics	Number in group	Calcium intake mg/d
Adults	not stated[311]	vegetarians who eat fish and chicken		
		- male	13	1122
		- female	24	840
		vegetarians who eat no animal flesh		
		- male	16	995
		- female	36	891
		vegetarians who eat no animal products (vegans)		
		- male	18	582
		- female	20	497
3 months old	1982[312]	Asian children aged 0-24 months (Indian and Pakistani)	54	414
6 months old			52	575
9 months old			47	798
12 months old			49	818
24 months old			47	783
Pregnant women	1977-80[308, 309]	All Asian pregnant women	813	1186
		Hindu vegetarian pregnant women	450	1253
		Hindu non-vegetarian pregnant women	225	1165
		Muslim non- vegetarian pregnant women	138	1002

9.10 Calcium intakes assessed using DRVs

9.10.1 Table 9.8 sets out the daily calcium intakes in relation to the DRVs. It is important to assess the dietary intakes of the group as a whole, without exclusions. The data from individuals with implausibly low energy intakes have therefore not been excluded. It is not appropriate to make assumptions that the dietary records from these individuals are necessarily inaccurate, particularly when no equivalent judgement can be made of the highest energy intakes.

Table 9.8 Mean daily calcium intakes† (mg) in Britain for specified population groups compared with the respective DRVs[287, 286, 288, 294]

Population Group	Mean calcium intake from food sources (mg)		RNI (mg/d)	Mean intakes expressed as % RNI		% of the group with intake below LRNI	
	Male	Female		Male	Female	Male	Female
1½ - 2½ years	682	643	350	195	184	<1	2
2½ - 3½ years	642	628	350	183	179	1	1
3½ - 4½ years*	625	595	450	139	132	2	3
10 - 11 years**	833	702	550	151	128	1	2
14 - 15 years	925	692	1000M/800F	93	87	5	18
16 - 24 years***	894	675	700	128	96	3	16
25 - 34 years	931	699	700	133	100	3	13
35 - 49 years	960	760	700	137	109	1	7
50 - 64 years	949	739	700	136	106	1	5
Not in institutions							
65 - 74 years	852	704	700	122	101	4	8
75 - 84 years	813	680	700	116	97	5	10
85+ years	764	647	700	109	92	2	15
Living in Institutions							
65 - 84 years	935	900	700	134	129	0	1
85+ years	981	828	700	140	118	1	1

Notes: † Table based on calcium derived from food sources only and excludes the contributions from supplements which were on average very small at all age groups

M= male; F = female

DRV = Dietary Reference Value; RNI = Reference Nutrient Intake; LRNI = Lower Reference Nutrient Intake

* DRV for 4-6 year olds used for assessment

** DRV for 7-10 year olds used for assessment

*** DRV for 19-50 year olds used for assessment

9.10.2 *Infants and preschool children*   The dietary intakes of calcium of infants aged 6-12 months are shown in Table 9.2 and para 9.4. These data are now over 10 years old. Mean values for calcium intake are close to 150 per cent of the RNI, and intake values at the extreme low end of the distribution are close to the RNI.   The quinquennial national surveys of infant feeding practices[313] do not quantitate nutrient intakes but they provide reassurance that the patterns of feeding infants in this country have not changed substantially in the past 10 years. Recent data are available on the calcium intakes of children aged 1½-4½ years (Table 9.2). These show that mean intakes are well above the RNI (Table 9.8). One per cent of children aged 1½-3½ years and 2 per cent of boys and 3 per cent of girls over 3½ years recorded intakes below the LRNI over the four day recording period.

In conclusion:

The calcium intakes of infants and children up to age 4½ years are adequate as assessed against the DRVs (conclusion 9.1.2).

9.10.3 *School children and adolescents* There is no recent national information about the nutrient intakes of school children in this country. A survey of diet and nutrition of young people aged 4-18 years in Britain completed fieldwork in early 1998 but no results are yet available. In 1983[294], a survey of 10-11 year olds found a mean daily intake of calcium for boys of 833mg and for girls of 702mg, compared with the RNI of 550mg for children aged 7-10 years and with the RNI for children aged 11-18 years of 1000mg for boys and 800mg for girls. Given that the RNI value for age 10-11 years is likely to lie between the values for the above age bands, these intakes appear adequate. One to two per cent of both the boys and the girls aged 10-11 years had intakes below the LRNI for children aged 7-10 years.

9.10.4 In the same survey, recorded mean calcium intakes of children aged 14-15 years were equivalent to 93 per cent of the RNI for boys and 87 per cent of the RNI for girls aged 11-18 years[294]. About 5 per cent of boys and about 18 per cent of girls recorded intakes below the LRNI. It is a matter of concern that this significant proportion had calcium intakes below those deemed to be adequate for the group as a whole. Another national survey in 1982[295] of 15-25 year olds found much higher calcium intakes than those recorded for these ages in other studies (Table 9.2). No estimates have been made of underreporting of dietary intakes in these studies and new data are urgently needed.

In conclusion:

There are no recent data about calcium intakes in primary school children. Data about older children are limited to specific ages and, because they were collected several years ago, may not reflect current dietary practices. It is not possible to draw firm conclusions for this age group but average intake was below RNI values in secondary school children, especially older girls, and all young people should take special care to avoid low calcium intakes. When the data from the National Diet and Nutrition Survey of young people are available, they should be reviewed with particular reference to calcium intakes and to identifying the characteristics of those whose intakes are low (conclusion 9.1.3).

9.10.5 *Women aged 16-64 years* National data for adults are now also over 10 years old[286] (para 9.4.5 and Table 9.2). Then, the mean daily calcium intake for women aged 16-24 years was 675mg which represents 84 per cent of the RNI for the 11-18 year age group and 96 per cent of the RNI for the age group aged 19 years and above. In the 25-34 year group of women the mean daily calcium intake was 699mg which equals the RNI, and similar values were recorded for older age groups. A significant proportion of women recorded calcium intakes below the LRNI of 400mg: 16 per cent at 16-24 years, 13 per cent at 25-34 years, 7 per cent at 35-49 years and 5 per cent at 50-64 years. Further analysis of the data showed evidence to suggest that the recorded intakes might not have represented habitual dietary practices, indicating some degree of underreporting. Of the total of 442 women aged 16-34 years, 220 reported food intake which contributed energy less than 1.2 calculated BMR. Virtually all of the individuals with intakes below LRNI were in this group. However, as 4 per cent of the women with energy intakes at or exceeding 1.2 BMR also had calcium intake levels below the LRNI, it would be difficult to justify ascribing values for calcium intake below the LRNI solely to deficiencies in the dietary records. The more prudent public health approach is to assume that a proportion of women, especially at younger ages have inadequate calcium intakes as judged by the DRV.

In conclusion:

The average calcium intakes of adult women are adequate compared to DRVs, although intakes of a proportion of women particularly in the younger groups are low. It is prudent for those with low calcium diets to increase their intakes. Underreporting may account for some of the apparent low intakes. A National Diet and Nutrition Survey of adults aged 19-64 years is now being planned to begin fieldwork in 1999 and should provide more up-to-date data from which calcium intake can be assessed (conclusion 9.1.4).

9.10.6   *Older women*   The mean calcium intakes of women over 50 years were close to the RNI value of 700mg which suggests that, on a group basis, calcium intakes are adequate. However, mean intake was below the RNI for women not living in institutions aged 75 years or older (Tables 9.2, 9.8). Of women aged 65 years or over not living in institutions 10 per cent recorded calcium intakes below the LRNI[288]. Although underreporting may have accounted for low recorded calcium intakes of a proportion of this group, it cannot be assumed that this accounts for the low calcium intakes in all cases. Women aged 65 years or over living in institutions, as a group, had mean calcium intakes above the RNI. Virtually no women in institutions recorded calcium intakes below the LRNI. This was attributed to the high proportion of milk and milk products in their diets.

In conclusion:

A proportion (less than 10 per cent) of older women in Britain not living in institutions appear to have calcium intake levels which are low as assessed against DRVs (conclusion 9.1.5).

9.10.7   *Pregnant and lactating women*   There are no national data for calcium intakes during pregnancy and lactation. The results from local surveys in pregnancy are recorded in Table 9.4 (para 9.4.7), and show adequate intakes in relation to the RNI of 700mg. Mean calcium intakes recorded during lactation are below the RNI of 1250mg for lactation (para 9.4.8) although intakes exceed the adult RNI value.

In conclusion:

There is no evidence that the diets of pregnant or lactating women do not provide adequate intakes of calcium (conclusion 9.1.6).

9.10.8 *Men*   At all ages the mean daily calcium intakes recorded for men exceeded the RNI value of 700mg (Table 9.8). The proportion of men aged 16-24 years with intakes below the LRNI was 3 per cent. For men not living in institutions aged 65 years or over, about 5 per cent recorded calcium intakes below the LRNI.

In conclusion:

In general, the calcium intakes for men appear to be adequate at all ages although there was a small proportion with intakes below the LRNI (conclusion 9.1.7).

10. Dietary intake and nutritional status of the population - vitamin D

10.1   Conclusions

10.1.1   **Children aged 0-3 years, pregnant and lactating women, and people aged 65 years or older, all of whom are vulnerable to vitamin D deficiency, had mean dietary intakes which were low.   The contribution from supplements, except in infants and young children, appears to be minimal and was lowest of all in groups of old people in institutions (para 10.9.4).**

10.1.2   **The vitamin D status, assessed from plasma 25(OH)vitamin D, of the majority of the population of children under 4 years appears to be satisfactory (para 10.9.1). Some minority groups of children remain at risk due to factors associated with lifestyle. The current programme of vitamin D supplementation for this section of the population should continue. Educational programmes to reinforce this policy appear to be needed (para 10.10.2).**

10.1.3   **There is no information about the vitamin D status, as assessed from 25(OH)vitamin D plasma levels of the UK population aged 4-64 years, nor of pregnant or lactating women. This will need to be reviewed urgently as the results of surveys now commissioned become available (para 10.10.4).**

10.1.4   **The vitamin D status of a significant minority of older people is low, particularly among those living in institutions. This nutritional deficiency is unsatisfactory for general health. It may also contribute to increasing the risk of fractures but further data from long term intervention trials are needed (para 10.10.7).**

10.2   Assessing vitamin D status

10.2.1   Both diet and sunlight contribute to the body's store of vitamin D. For most people, sunlight is the major factor in ensuring vitamin D adequacy, yet it cannot be quantified routinely. The dietary component is important for the whole population because of the limited period for synthesis from the skin. It is crucial for those who, for diverse reasons, do not expose their skin to sunlight.

10.2.2   The vitamin D status marker, plasma 25(OH)vitamin D, provides, for the first time, a means to assess vitamin D status in populations. The significance of different levels of this metabolite is being investigated (para 6.2.3). In considering the results of 25(OH)vitamin D values, the time of the year and the latitude of abode of the study participants need to be taken into account.

10.3   Dietary intakes of vitamin D of the British population

10.3.1   *Vitamin D intake from household foods*[285]   Most vitamin D is provided by margarine and other fat spreads (which are usually fortified), cereals (due to the fortification of some breakfast cereals with vitamin D), oily fish, meat, eggs and milk products (Table 10.1). The total amounts contributed by milk and milk products and by fats in the past 25 years show no significant trend although within these categories, there have been major shifts. Less is now obtained from whole milk and less from other milk and cream; while the amount from butter has also fallen, that from other fats (mainly reduced and low fat spreads) has increased (Table 10.2). Measurable amounts of vitamin D and its metabolites have now been found in carcase meat as a result of new analytical methods. The gradual introduction of these new data into the National Food Survey resulted in an increase in assessed vitamin D intake in 1995 and 1996 (Figure 10.1). For example, without the new meat data, vitamin D intake in 1995 would have been 2.69 µg/day with 1.1 per cent coming from meat and meat products but with the new data the intake is 2.96 µg/day with over 10 per cent coming from meat and meat products. Only oily fish, including herrings, tuna, salmon, sardines, mackerel, contribute significantly to vitamin D intake from fish. The proportion of vitamin D obtained from fish and fish products was 30 per cent in 1951; after a nadir in the 1980s, there has been a small increase in the 1990s (Table 10.3). The vitamin D density of the diet has gradually increased since 1975 (Figure 10.1).

Figure 10.1 Vitamin D content of British household food (1975-1996)

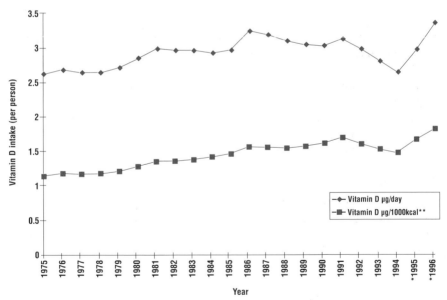

* the vitamin D content of food in 1995 and 1996 takes account of new analytical data on the amounts of vitamin D present in meat (see para 10.3.1)
** Vitamin D density of the diet
Source: MAFF, National Food Survey 1975-1996 (see para 8.1.1)

Table 10.1 Contributions made by selected foods to the vitamin D content of food purchased by British households - 1970-96 (average)

Food Source	Year													
	1970		1975		1980		1985		1990		1995		1996	
	µg/d	%	µg/d	%	µg/d	%	µg/d	%	µg/d	%	µg/d	%	µg/d	%
Total milk & milk products	0.26	9.2	0.36	13.5	0.25	8.7	0.32	11.0	0.26	8.7	0.23	7.8	0.23	6.9
- liquid whole milk	0.10	3.5	0.10	3.9	0.07	2.5	0.08	2.7	0.05	1.8	0.04	1.2	0.03	0.9
- dried milk skim	0.10	3.6	0.07	2.8	0.05	1.6	0.04	1.5	0.07	2.2	0.07	2.3	0.07	2.1
- other milk & cream	0.01	0.5	0.13	5.0	0.09	3.2	0.16	5.5	0.10	3.4	0.09	3.1	0.09	2.7
- cheese	0.05	1.7	0.05	1.9	0.04	1.4	0.04	1.3	0.04	1.3	0.04	1.2	0.04	1.2
Total Fats	1.22	42.6	1.14	43.3	1.39	48.9	1.49	50.3	1.52	50.2	1.26	42.5	1.30	38.8
- Butter	0.30	10.6	0.29	10.9	0.12	4.3	0.09	2.9	0.05	1.6	0.04	1.4	0.05	1.5
- Margarine	0.92	32.1	0.84	31.8	1.23	43.2	1.21	41.0	1.03	34.1	0.47	15.8	0.41	12.2
- All other fats	-	-	0.02	0.7	0.04	1.4	0.19	6.4	0.44	14.5	0.75	25.3	0.85	25.4
Eggs	0.50	17.4	0.44	16.9	0.46	16.2	0.35	11.7	0.28	9.3	0.24	7.9	0.24	7.2
Total Cereals	0.23	8.1	0.15	5.8	0.26	9.1	0.31	10.5	0.37	12.1	0.39	13.1	0.56	16.7
- "white" bread	-		-		-		-		-		-		-	
- other bread	-		-		-		-		-		0.01	0.4	0.01	0.3
- cakes, pastries, biscuits	0.12	4.1	0.08	3.2	0.06	2.3	0.07	2.2	0.03	0.9	0.03	1.1	0.04	1.2
- breakfast cereals	n/a		n/a		n/a		0.18	6.1	0.29	9.6	0.31	10.4	0.48	14.3
Total fruit & vegetables	-		-		-		-		-		0.01	0.4	0.01	0.3
Total meat & meat products	0.03	1.0	0.03	1.1	0.03	1.0	0.03	0.9	0.02	0.7	0.30	10.0	0.42	12.5
Total fish	0.57	20.0	0.48	18.4	0.42	14.9	0.44	14.9	0.56	18.4	0.51	17.3	0.55	16.4
Total beverages	0.04	1.2	0.02	0.7	0.03	1.1	0.02	0.7	0.01	0.4	0.01	0.4	0.01	0.3
Other foods	0.01	0.2	0.01	0.3	-		-		0.01	0.2	0.01	0.4	0.03	0.9
Total daily vitamin D intakes (µg)	2.87		2.63		2.85		2.96		3.02		2.96*		3.35*	

Notes: Figures may not add up due to rounding. n/a = data not available
* Since 1992 nutrients obtained from soft and alcoholic drinks and confectionery, and food and drink consumed outside the home have also been assessed.Soft and alcoholic drinks and confectionery, and food and drink consumed outside the home are excluded from the table but accounted for an extra 0.24µg vitamin D per day in 1995 and 0.23µg in 1996. The substantial increase in vitamin D from meat is a result of new

Table 10.2 Percentage contribution made by butter, margarine and other fats from 1955 to 1996 to the mean vitamin D content of household food in Britain (%)

Year	Butter	Margarine	Other fats	Total fats
1955	7.5	41.7	0.1	49.4
1960	10.6	36.2	0.3	47.1
1965	11.9	31.4	0.2	43.4
1970	10.6	32.1	-	42.6
1975	10.9	31.8	0.7	43.3
1980	4.3	43.2	1.4	48.9
1985	2.9	41.0	6.4	50.3
1990	1.6	34.1	14.5	50.2
1995	1.4	15.8	25.3	42.5
1996	1.3	12.2	25.3	38.9

Notes: Figures may not add up due to rounding.
Source: MAFF National Food Survey, 1955-96 (see para 8.1.1)

Table 10.3 Total and percentage contribution made by fish to the mean vitamin D content of household food in Britain (1955-96)

Year	Oily fish*		Other fish and fish products		Total fish	
	µg/d	%	µg/d	%	µg/d	%
1955	n/a	-	n/a	-	0.7	19.7
1960	0.33	9.7	0.50	15.4	0.83	25.1
1965	n/a	-	n/a	-	0.80	25.6
1970	0.52	18.1	0.05	1.8	0.57	20.0
1975	0.43	16.4	0.05	2.0	0.48	18.4
1980	0.42	14.6	0.01	0.3	0.42	14.9
1985	0.43	14.5	0.01	0.4	0.44	14.9
1990	0.54	17.9	0.02	0.6	0.56	18.4
1995	0.49	16.4	0.03	0.9	0.51	17.3
1996	0.52	15.6	0.03	0.9	0.55	16.5

Notes: n/a = data not available
* "oily fish" includes herring, tuna, sardine, salmon
Source: MAFF National Food Survey, 1955-96 (see para 8.1.1)

10.4   **Vitamin D intakes in specific population groups** (Table 10.4)

10.4.1   *Infants*   The total mean daily intake of vitamin D from food is higher at age 6-9 months (mean 4.70 µg/day) than at any other age. This can be attributed to drinking infant formula which has high levels of fortification. The 1986 survey of feeding practices in the second half of infancy reported a lower mean intake of vitamin D of 2.14 µg/day at age 9-12 months as mothers switched from infant formula to cows' milk[293]. More recent advice is that the introduction of cows' milk be delayed until 12 months of age. Formula milk is now being given for longer and as a result the vitamin D intakes of this age group are likely to have risen since 1986 (DH survey of 1997 - unpublished). For infants receiving them, vitamin D supplements contributed 63 per cent and 77 per cent of the total vitamin D intake at 6-9 months and 9-12 months respectively in 1986[293].

10.4.2   *Preschool children*   Mean intakes of vitamin D from all sources i.e. including supplements in children aged 1½-4½ years was 1.9µg/day of which supplements of vitamin D contributed somewhat less than about a half for all age groups. Children in the youngest age group (1½-2½ years) had significantly higher vitamin D intakes per 1000kcal energy intake than children in older age groups. In the youngest age group, much of the vitamin D came from 'other milk and milk products', which included infant formula, whereas in the oldest age group fat spreads and breakfast cereals, both of which are often fortified with vitamin D, were more important sources[287]. The mean daily intakes of vitamin D for children aged 1½-3½ years were slightly lower in 1992/3, than those recorded in 1967/8, but intakes at 3½-4½ years were comparable in the two surveys[287,289].

10.4.3   *Adults*   The Dietary and Nutritional Survey of British Adults found that men had an average intake of 3.78µg vitamin D per day, and women had an average intake of 3.09µg vitamin D per day, from all sources[286]. Of these intakes, supplements provided on average about 9 per cent for men and about 19 per cent for women. Intakes increased with age for both men and women. In this survey, most of the vitamin D from food was obtained from fats and fat spreads (30 per cent, mostly non-butter spreads), cereal products (24 per cent, mainly fortified breakfast cereals) and fish and fish dishes (22 per cent, mostly oily fish). The new vitamin D values for meat were not available at that time.

10.4.4   *Older adults*   From the age of 65 years mean intakes of vitamin D for men and women tended to decrease with age (Table 10.4). The intakes from all sources for men not living in institutions fell from 4.79 µg/day at 65-74 years to 4.27 µg/day at 75-84 years to 3.39 µg/day at 85 years and older, and matching mean intake levels for women were 3.51 µg/day at 65-74 years, 3.49 µg/day at 75-84 years and 2.89 µg/day at 85 years and over. Supplements (excluding prescribed supplements) contributed approximately 11 per cent of vitamin D intake in men and 15 per cent in women aged 65 years or over who were not living in institutions, but only contributed 1 per cent in those living in institutions. The contribution of fortified foods (fat spreads and breakfast cereals) to vitamin D intake was greater than that of supplements in this age group (estimated to be 37 per cent in men and 38 per cent in women). The recent survey of older people showed that current vitamin D intakes are higher[288] than had been recorded 22 years before[290]. The new methods to measure vitamin D in meat accounts for part but not all of the increase in intakes.

Table 10.4 Mean daily vitamin D intakes (µg) in Britain by age and sex

Age Group	Year of field work	Sex	Number in group	Mean vitamin D intake µg/d		
				total from all sources µg/d(1sd)	from food sources µg/d(1sd)	from supplements
6 - 9 months [293]	1986	Both	258	7.4	4.70 (4.79)	2.7
9 - 12 months [293]	1986	Both	230	4.2	2.14 (3.30)	2.1
6 - 18 months [289]	1967/8	Male Female	103 96	5.4* (n/a)	-	-
1½ - 2½ years [289]	1967/8	Male Female	186 181	2.9* (n/a)	-	-
2½ - 3½ years [289]	1967/8	Male Female	188 194	2.0* (n/a)	-	-
3½ - 4½ years [289]	1967/8	Male Female	164 142	1.8* (n/a)	-	-
1½ - 2½ years [287]	1992/3	Male Female	298 243	1.7 (2.1) 2.0 (2.3)	1.2 (1.2) 1.2 (1.1)	0.5 0.8
2½ - 3½ years [287]	1992/3	Male Female	350 306	1.7 (1.8) 1.9 (2.4)	1.2 (0.9) 1.2 (0.9)	0.5 0.7
3½ - 4½ years [287]	1992/3	Male Female	250 243	2.0 (2.3) 1.9 (2.1)	1.4 (1.1) 1.3 (0.8)	0.6 0.6
10 - 11 years [294]	1983	Male Female	902 821	1.48 (1.09) 1.32 (0.98)	-	-
14 - 15 years [294]	1983	Male Female	513 461	1.63 (1.30) 1.24 (0.89)	-	-
16 - 24 years [286]	1986/7	Male Female	214 189	3.02 (2.50) 2.44 (2.23)	2.81 (2.49) 2.10 (1.26)	0.21 0.34
25 - 34 years [286]	1986/7	Male Female	254 253	3.40 (2.61) 2.59 (2.22)	3.16 (2.31) 2.30 (1.57)	0.24 0.29
35 - 49 years [286]	1986/7	Male Female	346 385	4.17 (3.66) 3.20 (3.06)	3.71 (2.64) 2.61 (1.77)	0.46 0.59
50 - 64 years [286]	1986/7	Male Female	273 283	4.24 (3.78) 3.81 (3.63)	3.80 (2.80) 2.82 (2.07)	0.44 0.99
65 - 80 years [290] not in institutions	1972/3	Male Female	111 125	2.4 (1.64) 2.1 (1.79)	-	-
81+ years [290] not in institutions	1972/3	Male Female	58 71	2.7 (2.01) 2.3 (2.61)	-	-
65 - 74 years [288] not in institutions	1994/5	Male Female	271 256	4.79 (4.03)** 3.51 (2.93)**	4.25 (3.49)** 2.96 (2.54)**	0.54 0.55
75 - 84 years [288] not in institutions	1994/5	Male Female	265 217	4.27 (3.17)** 3.49 (2.85)**	3.81 (2.68)** 3.03 (2.40)**	0.46 0.46
65 - 84 years [288] living in institutions	1994/5	Male Female	128 91	3.65 (2.09)** 3.36 (1.81)**	3.62 (2.00)** 3.32 (1.83)**	0.03 0.04
85+ years [288] not in institutions	1994/5	Male Female	96 170	3.39 (2.43)** 2.89 (2.39)**	3.18 (2.19)** 2.31 (1.50)**	0.21 0.58
living in institutions		Male Female	76 117	4.22 (2.56)** 3.36 (1.76)**	4.08 (2.42)** 3.31 (1.76)**	0.14 0.05

Notes: large sd figures are due to a skew as a result of vitamin D supplementation.

n/a = data not available; sd = standard deviation

* data not available for males and females separately.

** includes data from new analyses of vitamin D in meat.

Older reports give mean values for total vitamin D intakes which include intakes from both food and supplements but values are not reported separately from these two sources.

10.5 Vitamin D intake attributable to fortification

10.5.1   The number of foods fortified with vitamin D has increased in the past 20 years and Government survey databases are regularly updated to take this into account. Some breakfast cereals and a few other foods, for example, reduced and low fat spreads and some yoghurts are now fortified voluntarily by the manufacturers, and such foods make an increasing contribution to vitamin D intake. Infant formula and manufactured weaning foods are both fortified with vitamin D and make a substantial contribution to the intakes of infants and young children. At older ages vitamin D from fortified breakfast cereals makes an increasing contribution. Within the non-butter fat spreads sector, margarine contributes a declining proportion and other fat spreads an increasing proportion (Table 10.2).

10.6 Contribution from dietary supplements to vitamin D intake

10.6.1   Only in infants do dietary supplements make a substantial contribution to the vitamin D intakes. In a recent national survey 23 per cent of mothers reported giving vitamin supplements to their babies at age about 14 months (Table 10.5) (Department of Health survey of 1997 - unpublished). During younger adult life, the proportion of intake from supplements tends to be low. Older people derive on average around 13 per cent of their intakes from supplements. The contribution made by supplements for those living in institutions is smallest of all.

Table 10.5 Proportion of babies receiving vitamin supplements in Britain by age - a comparison between the national population and a population of Asian origin (%)[313 314]

Age	Population Group			
	Pakistani	Bangladeshi	Indian	Nationally representative of UK
9 weeks	22	15	21	6
5 months	41	32	39	9
9 months	57	52	56	17
14/15 months	54	50	58	23
24 months	38	43	46	n/a

Notes: n/a = data not available

10.7 Variations in vitamin D intakes by region and income

10.7.1   The region with the highest intake was West Midlands and the lowest was Scotland as assessed from household foods, although the range of intakes from highest to lowest was narrow (about 0.5 µg/day)(Figure 10.2). As determined from surveys of individuals, total intakes were highest in London and South-East for preschool children which was probably due to higher intakes from vitamin supplements. At other ages there was no evidence of regional variation in intake (Table 10.6). Figure 10.3 shows vitamin D intakes, as assessed in the 1994-1996 National Food Survey by income group. It shows an increase in vitamin D intake with decreasing income.

Figure 10.2 Vitamin D content of British household food by region (1994-1996)

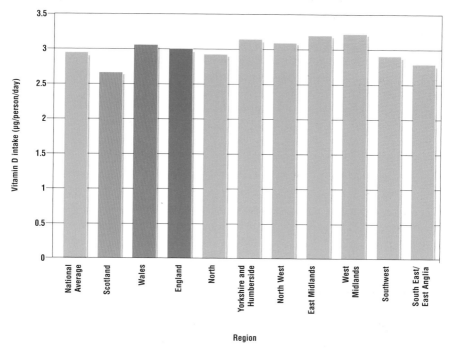

Source: MAFF, National Food Survey 1994-1996 (See Para 8.1.1)

Table 10.6 Mean daily vitamin D intakes (µg) from all sources (includes supplements), by age, sex and region of Britain

Age Group & Study	Sex	Number in group	Region			
			Scotland	England and Wales		
				Northern	Central, South-West & Wales	London and South-East
6 - 12 months[293]	Both	488	3.91	3.91	3.39	3.12
1½ - 4½ years[287]	Both	1675	1.4	1.7	1.9	2.2
10 - 11 years[294]	Male	1272*	1.24	1.54	1.54	1.40
	Female	1160*	1.15	1.36	1.40	1.24
14 - 15 years[294]	Male	512**	1.76	1.69	1.66	1.48
	Female	457**	1.09	1.33	1.27	1.14
16 - 64 years[286]	Male	1087	3.7	4.1	3.7	3.6
	Female	1110	2.8	3.3	2.9	3.3
65+ years [288] not in institutions	Male	632	4.40		4.96	4.23
	Female	643	3.13		3.53	3.67

Notes: * numbers differ from those in Table 10.4 as the regional analysis includes data from an additional Scottish sample.
　　　　** numbers differ slightly from those in Table 10.4 due to differences in regional analysis.

83

Figure 10.3 Vitamin D content of British household food by income group (1994-1996)

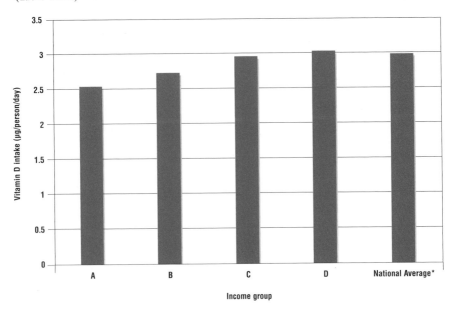

The level of income decreases from income group A to income group D
* National average also includes households without an earner and pensioner households.
Source: MAFF, National Food Survey 1994-1996 (See para 8.1.1)

10.8   The diets of minority groups

10.8.1   *Vegetarians*   Vegetarians who do not eat animal flesh had lower dietary intakes of vitamin D than people who ate fish and chicken (Table 10.7). Intakes of vitamin D from vegan diets were also lower.

10.8.2   *Diets from the Indian subcontinent*   Mean vitamin D intakes for Asian children at ages 6, 12 and 24 months were all substantially greater than the intakes recorded from the age matched general population (Table 10.7). The differences are likely to be due to higher intakes from vitamin supplements which are particularly encouraged for Asian under-fives. The rates of vitamin D supplement taking, up to the age of 2 years, are several times higher among children from Asian families.   While less than 20 per cent of a nationally representative population of infants and young children were receiving supplements, more than 50 per cent of Asian origin children were receiving them by the age of 9 months (Table 10.5). Information about the diets of Asian children up to age 2 years was obtained from a simple food frequency questionnaire. When compared with a group of white infants, Pakistani and Bangladeshi infants were more likely to be given cows' milk before age 1 year. At age 2 years 28 per cent of Indian children were vegetarian, 3 per cent of Bangladeshi, 4 per cent of Pakistani and 32 per cent of Indian children aged 2 years ate meat less than once a week or not at all[314]. Intakes of vitamin D in pregnancy from food sources were lower for Asian women than for white women, being lowest for vegetarian Asian women, for whom margarine was the major source[308,309].

84

Table 10.7 Mean daily vitamin D intakes (µg) of adult vegetarians and of young children and pregnant women from the Indian Subcontinent now living in Britain

Population Group	Year of fieldwork	Special characteristics	Number in group	Vitamin D intake µg/d
Adults	not stated[311]	vegetarians who eat fish and chicken - male - female	13 24	3.24 3.02
		vegetarians who eat no animal flesh - male - female	16 36	2.21 1.87
		vegetarians who eat no animal products (vegans) - male - female	18 20	1.87 1.58
3 months old	1982[312]	Asian children aged 0-24 months (Indian and Pakistani)	54	11.5
6 months old			52	12.3
9 months old			47	9.3
12 months old			49	12.4
24 months old			47	5.9
Pregnant women	1977-80 [309]	All Asian pregnant women	813	1.41
		Hindu vegetarian pregnant women	450	1.04
		Hindu non-vegetarian pregnant women	225	1.65
		Muslim non- vegetarian pregnant women	138	1.95

10.9   Vitamin D intakes assessed using DRVs

10.9.1   *Children aged 0-3 years*   Dietary vitamin D intake data from national surveys are shown in Table 10.4. The range of intakes is wide; mean intakes, which include supplements, are below the RNI at all ages except late infancy. Particular groups in the population are more vulnerable to deficiency (para 6.2.14) and educational programmes have, for many years, advised health professionals about how to identify infants and children under 5 years who might particularly benefit from vitamin D supplements. It is not known whether the children with high intakes in the survey were from groups that were most vulnerable but there is anecdotal evidence of successful targeting. The results from recent surveys suggest that more Asian preschool children are being advised to take vitamin supplements (including vitamin D) than white children (Table 10.5).

10.9.2   *Children, adolescents and adults*   There are no DRVs for vitamin D for ages 4-64 years on the basis that the requirements are met from skin synthesis. There is a limited contribution from the diet with a mean of 1-2 µg daily in school children, which rises to daily mean intakes of 2-4 µg in adult groups (Table 10.4). These data are taken from surveys in the 1980s. There will be more up-to-date information when the results of current surveys of this population group are published. These data should be reviewed as soon as they are available.

10.9.3   Vulnerable groups who may not achieve a satisfactory status are advised to take daily supplements of 10 µg vitamin D. These include those who do not expose their skin to sunlight for a variety of reasons (para 6.2.9) and some ethnic minority groups especially if they have pigmented skin and choose diets which exclude meat and fish. There are no data about the vitamin D intakes of these vulnerable groups such as women who conceal themselves at all times when out of doors. This lifestyle has been associated with an inadequate vitamin D status in other countries. Pregnant women are also recognised as vulnerable because they need to provide vitamin D for the fetus, as are lactating women who need to replenish their own stores of vitamin D. There are limited data about the intakes of vitamin D during pregnancy which suggest they do not differ from the intakes of non-pregnant women and therefore do not meet the RNI.

10.9.4   *Older adults*   In spite of this increasing vulnerability, mean total vitamin D intakes, whether from food or from dietary supplements did not exceed 5 µg/day and the levels of intake fell with age.

In conclusion:

Children aged 0-3 years, pregnant and lactating women, and people aged 65 years or older, all of whom are vulnerable to vitamin D deficiency, had mean dietary intakes which were low. The contribution from supplements, except in infants and young children appears to be minimal, and was lowest of all in groups of old people in institutions (conclusion 10.1.1).

10.10   Nutritional status assessed from plasma 25(OH)vitamin D

10.10.1   *Preschool children*   The National Diet and Nutrition Survey of children aged 1½-4½ years measured plasma 25(OH)vitamin D levels (Table 10.8)[287]. Group mean levels were around 65-70nmol/l, and individual levels for almost all children were above 25nmol/l, the value chosen to denote adequate vitamin D status although two out of a total of 737 children had levels of 15nmol/l (6 µg/l). The seasonal variation in levels of 25(OH)vitamin D in the plasma was confirmed (Fig 10.4).

10.10.2   *Two year olds from Asian families in the UK*   A nationally representative sample of preschool children includes only few children from the ethnic minority groups. Thus, unless the survey is very large, there would be too few children from these groups for separate analysis of results. For this reason, and because 2 year olds from Asian families are thought to be vulnerable, a separate survey was done in 1996. Table 10.8 shows the mean plasma 25(OH)vitamin D levels for 2 year old children born in this country to families originally from Pakistan, India and Bangladesh. All the blood samples from the Asian 2 year olds were taken in November which is a time when stores should still have been available if the young child is to survive the winter without becoming deficient. It is therefore a matter of concern that 34 per cent of Pakistani, 25 per cent of Indian and 20 per cent of Bangladeshi young children had values below 25nmol/l (10 µg/l)[315]. Dietary factors which were particularly associated with low 25(OH)vitamin D status were not being given vitamin supplements, evidence of iron deficiency with low haemoglobin and low ferritin, and consumption of chapati. Other factors

Figure 10.4 Mean plasma 25-hydroxyvitamin D levels (nmol/l) in children aged 1½ to 4½ years, people aged 65 years and over, by season (representative British population)

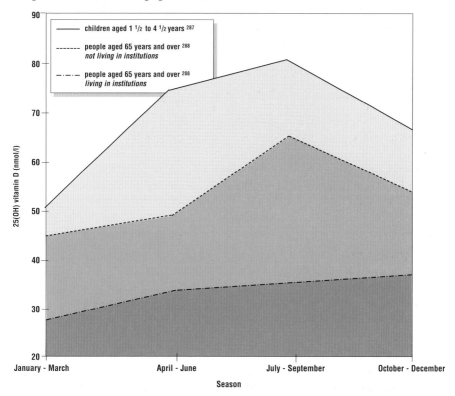

which showed a trend, but not of statistical significance, were giving cows' milk at or before 9 months of age and high intake of cows' milk at 2 years.

The vitamin D status, assessed from plasma 25(OH)vitamin D, of the majority population of children under 4 years appears to be satisfactory (para 10.9.1). Some minority groups of children remain at risk due to factors associated with lifestyle. The current programme of vitamin D supplementation for this section of the population should continue. Educational programmes to reinforce this policy appear to be needed (conclusion 10.1.2).

10.10.3 *School children and younger adults*   There is no information about the 25(OH)vitamin D levels of the nationally representative population of school children and adults up to age 64 years in the UK. These data have been included in national surveys which are now being conducted (Annex 3). More information is urgently needed about vulnerable minority groups in the population (para 10.9.3).

Table 10.8 Plasma 25(OH)vitamin D levels in British children aged 1½-4½ years[287] and in two year olds in England in families originally from Bangladesh, India and Pakistan[315]

Population group and age	Date of fieldwork	Number in group	Mean plasma 25(OH) vitamin D, nmol/l (one sd) [µg/l, (one sd)]	Percentage of group with 25(OH) vitamin D below:				
				12.5 nmol/1	20 nmol/1	25 nmol/1	50 nmol/1	75 nmol/1
				%	%	%	%	%
British population 1½ - 2½ years	1992/3*	213	67.4(21.8) [27.0(8.7)]	0	1	1	17	64
British population 2½ - 3½	1992/3*	274	66.6.(21.6)[26.6(8.6)]	0	1	1	23	62
British population 3½ - 4½	1992/3*	120(M) 130(F)	70.1(19.4)[28.0(78)] 70.3(21.6)[28.1(8.6)]	0 0	0 0	0 0	12 22	58 58
Bangladeshi origin 2 years	November 1996	139	42.1(21.3)[16.8(8.5)]	0	13	20	69	91
Indian origin 2 years	November 1996	279	42.2(22.5)[16.9(9)]	0	13	25	70	89
Pakistani origin 2 years	November 1996	200	36.2(19.6)[14.5(7.8)]	0	18	34	81	95

Notes: * Fieldwork evenly spread across 12 months
        M = male
        F = female
        sd = standard deviation

10.10.4 *Pregnant and lactating women*   There are no national data about the vitamin D status of pregnant or lactating women in the UK. In Cardiff, 32 Asian and 63 Caucasian women in early pregnancy had blood sampled for plasma PTH. Of 12 Asians with raised PTH concentrations all those measured (9) had very low plasma 25(OH)vitamin D, in two cases the values were below 2.5nmol/l(1.0 µg/l). None of the Caucasian women had low plasma 25(OH)vitamin D[14].

In conclusion:

There is no information about the vitamin D status, as assessed from 25(OH)vitamin D plasma levels of the UK population aged 4-64 years, nor of pregnant or lactating women. This will need to be reviewed urgently as the results of surveys now commissioned become available (conclusion 10.1.3).

10.10.5 *Older adults*   The plasma 25(OH)vitamin D levels in people older than 65 years has been assessed in a large British study which spanned a 12 month period[288]. The participants were grouped according to whether they lived in an institution or not (see Table 10.9). The mean plasma 25(OH)vitamin D level declined with increasing age especially in the over 85s. Women tended to have lower levels than men, and the levels for both sexes were substantially lower where people were resident in institutions (Fig 10.4). The proportions of the groups with plasma 25(OH)vitamin D levels below arbitrary cut-off levels also reflects these trends. Seasonal differences between summer and winter were recorded for all groups except the group of elderly institutionalised people who had the same vitamin D status in summer as in winter which, in a proportion of the group, was inadequate. This lack of boost to vitamin D status from summer sunshine suggests that these individuals relied entirely on diet for their intakes. A significant proportion of the very elderly population not living in institutions had plasma 25(OH)vitamin D concentrations below 25nmol/l, and the proportion was higher in those living in institutions where 37 per cent of residents had an inadequate status judged by this criterion.

Table 10.9 Plasma levels of 25(OH)vitamin D in British adults aged 65+ years[288]

Age group & study	Year* of fieldwork	Sex	Number in group	Mean plasma 25(OH)vitamin D, nmol/l, (one sd) [µg/l(one sd)]	Percentage of group with 25(OH) vitamin D below:						
					10 nmol/l	15 nmol/l	20 nmol/l	25 nmol/l	30 nmol/l	40 nmol/l	60 nmol/l
					%	%	%	%	%	%	%
65 - 74 years *not in institution*	1994/5	Male	212	63.7(30.0) [25.5(12.0)]	0	1	3	5	10	17	51
		Female	186	54.6(25.1) [21.8(10.0)]	0	0	4	6	16	37	64
75 - 84 years *not in institution*	1994/5	Male	196	54.7(24.9) [21.9(9.9)]	2	3	3	5	11	33	64
		Female	155	49.7(24.0) [19.9(9.6)]	1	5	7	15	24	39	67
85 + years *not in institution*	1994/5	Male	68	46.7(23.1) [18.7(9.2)]	0	3	9	13	22	46	78
		Female	110	41.5(21.5) [16.6(8.6)]	2	4	15	25	31	55	84
65 - 84 years *living in institution*	1994/5	Male	84	33.6(15.3) [13.4(6.1)]	2	5	17	36	51	69	94
	1994/5	Female	58	34.1(17.0) [13.6(6.8)]	0	4	18	38	47	75	89
85 + years *living in institution*	1994/5	Male	54	34.0(17.8) [13.6(7.1)]	2	11	22	42	53	68	90
	1994/5	Female	62	30.8(13.5) [12.3(5.4)]	2	5	19	36	53	86	94

Notes: *Fieldwork evenly spread across 12 months
                  sd = standard deviation

10.10.6 The seasonal effect on vitamin D status is shown in Figure 10.4. The available information from published papers about the seasonal variation in plasma 25(OH)vitamin D levels in the UK has been collated in Table 10.10. While one study is not necessarily directly comparable with another because of assay modifications over 25 years, the within study comparisons confirm the declining status with age. For older people living in institutions there is evidence of vitamin D insufficiency in a significant proportion. Further, there is no boost in vitamin D status in the summer months which is compatible with being housebound. This lack of a seasonal variation in this group is demonstrated also in Figure 10.4.

10.10.7 Elderly people are at considerable risk of vitamin D insufficiency which may lead to secondary hyperparathyroidism and bone loss especially during the winter. A proportion of people who are housebound or who live in institutions appear to be deficient in vitamin D throughout the whole year. Even when satisfactory vitamin D status is achieved for the summer months, there is a risk that bone loss incurred during the previous winter will not be regained in full leading to an incremental deterioration in bone health.

In conclusion:

The vitamin D status of a significant minority of older people is low particularly among those living in institutions. This nutritional deficiency is unsatisfactory for general health. It may also contribute to increasing the risk of fractures but further data from long term intervention trials are needed (conclusion 10.1.4).

Table 10.10 Seasonal variations in plasma 25(OH)vitamin D levels in the UK in healthy white populations (collated studies reported in past 25 years)

Age and circumstance	Sex	Number in group	Season	Mean plasma 25(OH)vitamin D (nmol/l)
1$\frac{1}{2}$ - 4$\frac{1}{2}$ years[287]	M + F	168 194	July - Sept Jan - March	80.1(sd 19.8) 51.0(sd 16.0)
4$\frac{1}{2}$ - 6$\frac{1}{2}$ years[316]	M+F	110	Aug Feb	53.0(sd 21.2) 27.8(sd 11.1)
12 - 17 years[164] 14 - 17 years[164]	M F	59 15	Sept - Oct Jan	56.5(33.5-94.7 95% ci) 32.3(18.0-58.0 95% ci)
18 - 37 years[164] 18 - 37 years[164]	M + F M + F	27 19	Oct - Nov March	53.3(27.0-104.4 95% ci) 32.3(16.5-63.0 95% ci)
24 - 45 years[165]	M + F	11	Sept March	90.5 (sd 23.0) 66.7(sd 17.7)
65 - 74 years[155] *healthy volunteers*	M + F	96*	Sept - Oct March - April	35.4(sd 11.5) 22.7(sd 10.8)
65 + years[288] *not in institution*	M + F	215 194	July - Sept Jan - March	64.8(sd 27.6) 45.0(sd 22.9)
65 + years [288] *living in institution*	M + F	54 52	July - Sept Jan - March	35.4(sd 18.2) 28.1(sd 14.6)
72 - 86 years[166] *healthy living at home*	M + F	19* 23*	July - Aug Dec - Feb	25.3(2.2 se of mean) 8.8(1.1 se of mean)
70 - 88 years *healthy* [317]	M + F	36*	Sept Dec - Jan	35.3(sd 12.25) 21.5(sd 7.7)
68 - 82 years[318] *attending day hospital*	M + F	10*	Sept March	5.5(2.9-10.5 95% ci) 7 (3.1-15.8 95% ci)
living in institution		77*	Sept March	5.8 (3.2-10.7 95% ci) 6.6 (3.5-12.4 95% ci)

Notes: *Longitudinal study(other studies measured individuals once only)
sd = standard deviation
ci = confidence intervals
se = standard error

11. Conclusions and recommendations

We recommend that:

1. A healthy lifestyle to maintain bone health should be encouraged at all ages. A varied and adequate diet and regular weight bearing physical activity appropriate for the individual are beneficial. An adequate vitamin D status can be achieved from exposure of the skin to summer sunlight although this needs to be balanced against increasing the risk of skin cancer. Local public health policies should integrate these recommendations in their plans for improving the health of their population[3,4].

11.1 The UK diet and bone health

11.1.1 *The DRVs for calcium* (para 5.3)   It is important to be aware of the limitations inherent in setting DRVs for calcium. The factorial approach, which involves a theoretical calculation of the requirements for calcium for growth and maintenance, needs to take into account the uncertainties of dietary bioefficacy. There are no intermediate markers of nutritional status for calcium: plasma ionised calcium is highly conserved, and other blood or urine markers have not been validated. In reviewing the DRVs for calcium, the Subgroup could find no evidence to support a change in the method of calculating DRVs from that used in 1991[17]. Using markers of bone status, as indicators of calcium nutritional status, such as that adopted by the USA NIH Consensus Panel[15], was rejected because of absence of evidence relating habitual calcium intake to bone outcomes. In reviewing the calcium DRVs set for the UK in 1991 for population age/gender groups, none of the scientific data were persuasive in leading to suggestions for changes. Only the increment for lactation has been difficult to justify and, if further data are supportive, a reduction in this value might be appropriate in the future. Particular attention was addressed to the RNI for postmenopausal women. The data do not show evidence of long term benefits to the health of this population group as a whole from dietary intakes above those of the UK RNI, although in cases of established osteoporosis, supplemental calcium might have a role as one part of a therapeutic strategy.

We recommend that:

2. There is insufficient evidence to recommend a change in the existing UK Dietary Reference Values for calcium. Recent data do not support the increment for lactation which might not be necessary.

11.1.2 *The DRVs for vitamin D* (para 6.3)   For the majority of the population, the diet does not contribute the major portion of metabolically available vitamin D and, as a result, establishing an RNI for vitamin D presents uncertainties. In some countries, for instance, Australia, no DRVs for vitamin D are set. In the United Kingdom, where opportunities for skin synthesis are limited by the northerly latitude and other risk factors are common, the contribution from the diet and from supplements can be relatively important particularly in vulnerable subgroups of the population. Plasma 25(OH)vitamin D and plasma PTH levels, provide intermediate markers as indicators of vitamin D status. The 1991 DRVs for vitamin D for infants, pregnant and lactating mothers and people over 65 years were confirmed. If the recommendations designed to reduce the risk of skin cancer so constrain the opportunities for skin synthesis of vitamin D that the risk of deficiency becomes general, the DRVs may need to be reviewed especially in groups where there is now no RNI.

We recommend that:

3. The existing UK Dietary Reference Values for vitamin D are endorsed.

11.2   The nutritional adequacy for calcium and vitamin D of the UK population

11.2.1   *Calcium dietary intakes* (para 9.3, 9.4)   Nutritional adequacy for calcium is best assessed as habitual intake relative to the DRVs for the UK. On this basis the majority of each population group appears to have an adequate calcium intake although the data are limited. Up-to-date representative data about school children will be available in 1999 and about adults aged 19-64 years in 2002. The available information suggests that 10-15 per cent of adolescents, younger women and women over 75 years not in institutions are consuming diets which provide calcium intakes which do not meet LRNI levels and therefore their intakes at this low level may not be adequate for optimal bone health in this country. For men not living in institutions aged 65 years or over, about 5 per cent recorded calcium intakes below the LRNI.

11.2.2   *Vitamin D dietary intakes* (para 10.3, 10.4)   Assessing dietary intakes of vitamin D against the RNI is only relevant for a limited number of population groups, (under 4 year olds, 65 year olds and older, and pregnant and lactating women) because no RNI is set for all other ages. In all groups except infants aged 6-9 months the average intakes (including those from supplements) were well below the RNI values. This does not necessarily imply that the nutritional status for vitamin D was unsatisfactory provided there was an opportunity for skin synthesis of vitamin D from moderate exposure to sunlight. It was recognised that although there are no vitamin D dietary values for most children and adults under 65 years, within this group a small minority with particular risk factors for vitamin D deficiency continue to rely significantly on an oral intake which is more reliably obtained from supplements. There are no reports to suggest that this vulnerable group is being identified or advised appropriately about the importance of preventing vitamin D deficiency. It is important that the general public and those responsible for developing public health policies, should be better informed about the difficulties of maintaining an adequate vitamin D status at UK latitudes, how to identify risk factors, and when to advise vitamin D supplements. Community based campaigns of education and promotion may be indicated such as the "Stop Rickets" campaign in the 1980s. Further consideration should be given to developing a national policy on exposure to sunlight to take account of the benefit of self-synthesis of vitamin D and the adverse effect on skin in regard to the risk of skin cancer.

11.2.3 *Vitamin D nutritional status* (para 10.2)   The vulnerable groups for vitamin D deficiency are those who, for one reason or another, are thought unlikely to synthesise sufficient vitamin D in their skin to meet their needs and in whom dietary intake is therefore critical. Population data to assess vitamin D status from plasma 25(OH)vitamin D levels are scarce and data using plasma PTH levels, more so. The limited number of studies has tended to focus on high risk groups and there is no evidence about other groups. The Subgroup found evidence of marginal or low vitamin D status in a significant minority of people of various ages, not only amongst the accepted vulnerable groups. Deficiency of vitamin D which leads to clinical rickets and osteomalacia still occurs sporadically as does the possibility of marginal vitamin D status. These findings endorse the importance of achieving the RNI for the vulnerable groups in the population, if necessary through supplementation.

We recommend that:

4. Local health authorities and health professionals should be aware that sporadic cases of clinical vitamin D deficiency still occur. They should be alert to the possibilities of inadequacies in their population from knowledge of the social and cultural antecedents of vitamin D deficiency and should consider instituting appropriate community-based preventive programmes.

11.3   Ensuring adequate calcium and vitamin D status for bone health

11.3.1 *Dietary means*   The best way of ensuring that nutritional status for calcium and for vitamin D are adequate for bone health is to integrate these requirements in the patterns for healthy living and eating set out in Eight Guidelines for a Healthy Diet[235] and the Balance of Good Health[319]. Calcium intakes for the majority of the population should not fall below those currently being recorded and intakes should increase for those with the lowest intakes. The household foods which contribute calcium to the British diet are shown in Table 9.1. Annex 4 (Table A4.1) lists the calcium content of portion sizes of some foods. While calcium intakes have declined by some 15 per cent in the past 25 years, the proportionate contributions from different foods remain similar. Thus, milk and milk products have consistently contributed some 60 per cent, and cereals about 25 per cent, while other food groups make a more limited contribution. Healthy eating policies promote increased bread consumption which favours an increase in calcium intakes provided fortification is retained (see below). Skimmed or semi-skimmed milk, which has the same calcium content as whole milk, is preferred so as not to increase the intake of fat, and it is encouraging to see the comparative increase in this market segment. The vitamin D intake from household foods purchased in Britain comes mainly from fortified foods, particularly margarine and spreading fats, and breakfast cereals (Table 10.1). Oily fish, (but not white fish) (Table 10.3) and meat, which are the major foods naturally rich in vitamin D, together make a contribution of something over 25 per cent. Oily fish have particularly been endorsed as contributing to a diet to promote cardiovascular health. Meat at moderate intakes makes an important contribution of several nutrients. The calcium and vitamin D content in portions of some foods are listed in Annex 4 (Table A4.2).

11.3.2 *Food fortification* Calcium added compulsorily to flour contributes 12-14 per cent of the total intake and without this proportion, the intakes of many more individuals would fall below DRVs. Calcium fortification of bread should therefore be retained. Bread is a major component in the diets of children and older people; both are groups where it is important to ensure that calcium intakes do not fall below current levels. Although the bread consumption of younger adults is less than formerly, it remains an important dietary component, and there is no alternative food that might have a wider uptake than bread. Continued compulsory fortification of margarine with vitamin D and the voluntary fortification of other fat spreads and of breakfast cereals with vitamin D should be continued.

11.3.3 *Dietary supplements* Calcium supplements have no demonstrable role in public health policies to improve bone health, although they may be useful therapeutically. Vitamin D supplementation is the only realistic means of achieving the RNI values for most people who rely on a dietary source as their major safeguard for achieving an adequate vitamin D status. There needs to be an increase in the low rates of vitamin D supplement taking in the at risk groups, especially during the winter months. Some groups, especially those from Asian communities or older people especially those who are housebound or who seldom go out of doors[320], need supplements all year round.

We recommend that:

5. Dietary means of achieving an adequate calcium intake, as assessed against Dietary Reference Values, should be encouraged.

We recommend that:

6. The present policy of fortifying flour with calcium should continue.

We recommend that:

7. The public and health professionals should be better informed about the importance of achieving adequate vitamin D status, including the appropriate use of vitamin supplements for those most at risk of vitamin D deficiency. The most vulnerable groups include:

- **infants, young children and pregnant women from Asian families as well as young African-Caribbean children being reared on strict exclusion diets;**

- **older people who are housebound, who live in institutions or who eat no meat or oily fish;**

- **and people who rarely go out of doors or who, when they do so, wear clothes which fully conceal them.**

We recommend that:

8. The statutory requirement to fortify margarine with vitamin D should be maintained; reduced fat spreads should also be fortified with vitamin D but

providing the majority of manufacturers continue to do this on a voluntary basis there is no need for this to be a statutory requirement.

11.4 Maintaining a healthy bodyweight

Being underweight is undesirable at any age and osteoporosis is more likely if individuals are of low body weight, although osteoporosis also occurs, but less commonly, in people who are overweight. A diet which is inadequate in energy is often also deficient in nutrients. Ensuring that a well balanced adequate diet is consumed is important in helping to maintain bone health.

We recommend that:

9. Maintenance of a healthy body weight at all ages should be encouraged. Being underweight is particularly detrimental to bone health.

11.5 Physical activity

Physical activity is an important lifestyle factor which should be included in public health policies to promote improved health. In this country physical activity levels have probably declined over several years in all sections of the population[321]. Weight bearing physical activity in children and younger adults helps to ensure optimal peak bone mass (although prolonged and strenuous activity seen with professional dancing or repeated strenuous jogging sometimes has the opposite effect). It is probable that physical activity levels distinguish populations at high risk of fracture in the Western developed world from those at low risk of fracture in developing countries. At older ages even the most frail can benefit from a more active life provided the activity is appropriate to the individual. Although the types of physical activity appropriate for old people may not be vigorous enough to give demonstrable changes in bone mass, they improve muscle tone and reduce the risk of falls as well as helping to maintain cardiovascular health.

We recommend that:

10. A lifestyle which includes regular physical activity, particularly that which is weight bearing, should be encouraged at all ages, and a sedentary lifestyle discouraged.

12. References

[1] Department of Health. *Advisory Group on Osteoporosis.* London: Department of Health, 1994.

[2] Royal College of Physicians. *Clinical Guidelines for Strategies to Prevent and Treat Osteoporosis.* London: Royal College of Physicians, (in press).

[3] Department of Health. *Our Healthier Nation: a contract for health.* Command paper 3852. London: The Stationery Office, 1998.

[4] The Scottish Office. *Working Together for a Healthier Scotland.* Command paper 3854. Edinburgh: The Stationery Office, 1998.

[5] Royal College of Physicians. *Fractured Neck of Femur.* London: Royal College of Physicians, 1989.

[6] Grimley Evans J, Seagroatt V, Goldacre MJ. Secular trends in proximal femoral fracture, Oxford record linkage study area and England 1968-86. *J Epidemiol Community Health* 1997; **51**:424-9.

[7] Melton LJ, Atkinson EJ, Madhok R, Robbins J. Downturn in hip fracture incidence. *Public Health Reports* 1996; **111**:146-51.

[8] Chick H, Dalyell EJ, Hume EM, Mackay HMM, Henderson Smith H, Wimberger H. Studies of rickets in Vienna: 1919-1922; report of the Accessory Food Factors Committee. *Medical Research Council Special Report Series No 77.* London: HMSO, 1923.

[9] James JA, Clark C, Ward PS. Screening Rastafarian children for nutritional rickets. *BMJ* 1985; **290**:899-900.

[10] Mughal MZ, Salama H, Greenaway T, Laing I, Mawer EB. Florid rickets associated with prolonged breast-feeding and maternal vitamin D deficiency: case reports. *BMJ* (in press).

[11] Department of Health and Social Security. *Rickets and Osteomalacia.* Report on Health and Social Subjects: 19. London: HMSO, 1980.

[12] Dunnigan MG, Glekin BM, Henderson JB, McIntosh WB, Sumner D, Sutherland GR. Prevention of rickets in Asian children: assessment of the Glasgow campaign. *BMJ* 1985; **291**:239-42.

[13] Iqbal SJ, Garrick DP, Howl A. Evidence of continuing "deprivational" vitamin D deficiency in Asians in the UK. *J Hum Nutr Diet* 1994; **7**:47-52.

[14] Alfaham M, Woodhead S, Pask G, Davies D. Vitamin D deficiency: a concern in pregnant Asian women. *Br J Nutr* 1995; **73**:881-7.

[15] National Institutes of Health Consensus Development Panel. Optimal Calcium Intake. *JAMA* 1994; **272**:1942-8.

[16] National Research Council (U.S.). Subcommittee on the Tenth Edition of the RDAs. *Recommended dietary allowances.* Food and Nutrition Board, Commission on Life Sciences. National Research Council, 10th rev. ed. Washington, D.C.: National Academy of Life Sciences, 1989.

[17] Department of Health. *Dietary Reference Values for Food Energy and Nutrients for the United Kingdom*. Report on Health and Social Subjects: 41. London: HMSO, 1991.

[18] Department of Health. *The Fortification of Yellow Fats with Vitamins A and D*. Report on Health and Social Subjects: 40. London: HMSO, 1991.

[19] Ministry of Agriculture, Fisheries and Food. *Food Standards Committee Second Draft on Bread and Flour*. London: HMSO, 1974.

[20] Department of Health and Social Security. *Nutritional Aspects of Bread and Flour*. Report on Health and Social Subjects: 23. London: HMSO, 1981.

[21] Iqbal SJ, Kaddam I, Wassif W, Nichol F, Walls J. Continuing clinically severe vitamin D deficiency in Asians in the UK (Leicester). *Postgrad Med J* 1994; **70**: 708-14.

[22] Finch PJ, Ang L, Eastwood JB, Maxwell JD. Clinical and histological spectrum of osteomalacia among Asians in South London. *Q J Med* 1992; **302**:439-48.

[23] Train JJA, Yates RW, Sury MRJ. Hypocalcaemic stridor and infantile nutritional rickets. *BMJ* 1995; **310**:48-9.

[24] Dunnigan MG, McIntosh WB, Sutherland GR, Gardee R, Glekin B, Ford JA, Robertson I. Policy for prevention of Asian rickets in Britain: a preliminary assessment of the Glasgow rickets campaign. *BMJ* 1981; **282**:357-60.

[25] Grindulis H, Scott PH, Bolton NR, Wharton BA. Combined efficiency of iron and vitamin D in Asian toddlers. *Arch Dis Child* 1986; **61**:843-8.

[26] Kanis JA. (a) Calcium nutrition and its implications for osteoporosis. Part I: Children and healthy adults. *Eur J Clin Nutr* 1994; **48**:757-67.

[27] Kanis JA. (b) Calcium nutrition and its implications for osteoporosis. Part II: After menopause. *Eur J Clin Nutr* 1994; **48**:833-41.

[28] Parfitt AM. Morphological basis of bone mineral measurements: transient and steady state effects of treatment in osteoporosis. *Miner Electrolyte Metab* 1980; **4**:273-87.

[29] Heaney RP. The bone-remodeling transient: implications for the interpretation of clinical studies of bone mass change. *J Bone Min Res* 1994; **9**:1515-23.

[30] Brown EM, Pollack M, Seidman CE, Seidman JG, Chou YHW, Riccardi D, Hebert SC. Calcium-ion sensing cell-surface receptors. *N Engl J Med* 1995; **333**:234-40.

[31] Zeghoud F, Vervel C, Guillozo H, Walraut-Debray O, Boutignon H, Garabédian M. Subclinical vitamin D deficiency in neonates: definition and response to vitamin D supplements. *Am J Clin Nutr* 1997; **65**:711-8.

[32] Khaw KT, Scragg R, Murphy S. Single dose cholecalciferol suppresses the winter increase in parathyroid hormone concentrations in normal older men and women: a randomized trial. *Am J Clin Nutr* 1994; **59(5)**:1040-4.

[33] Clements MR, Johnson L, Fraser DR. A new mechanism for induced vitamin D deficiency in calcium deprivation. *Nature* 1987; **324**:62.

[34] Pettifor JM. Dietary calcium deficiency. In: FH Florieux, ed. Rickets. New York: Raven press 1991, pp123-144.

[35] Jubiz W, Canterbury JM, Reiss JM, Tyler FM. Circadian rhythm in serum parathyroid hormone concentrations in human subjects: correlation with serum calcium, phosphate, albumin and growth hormone levels. *J Clin Invest* 1972; **51**:2040-6.

[36] Logue FC, Fraser WD, O'Reilly DstJ, Beastall GH. The circadian rhythm of intact parathyroid hormone and nephrogenous cyclic adenosine monophosphate in normal men. *J Endocrinol* 1989; **121**:R1-R3.

[37] Calvo MS, Kumar R, Heath III H. Elevated secretion and action of serum parathyroid hormone in young adults consuming high phosphorous, low calcium diets assembled from common foods. *J Clin Endocrinol Metab* 1988; **66**:823-9.

[38] Fraser WD, Logue FC, Christie JP, Gallacher SJ, Cameron D, O'Reilly DstJ, Beastall GH, Boyle IT. Alternation of the circadian rhythm of intact parathyroid hormone and serum phosphate in women with established post menopausal osteoporosis. *Osteoporos Int* 1998; **8/2**:121-126.

[39] Reeve J, Davies UM, Hesp R, McNally E, Katz D. Treatment of osteoporosis with human parathyroid peptide and observations on effect of sodium fluoride. *BMJ* 1990; **301**:314-8.

[40] Black AJ, Charlwood C, Durham B, Fraser WD. Timed therapy with calcium and phosphate supplements restores phosphate and parathyroid hormone rhythms in patients with osteoporosis with an anabolic effect on spinal bone mineral density. *Br J Rheumatol* 1996; **35**(suppl 1): Abstract 167.

[41] World Health Organisation. Assessment of Fracture Risk and its application to screening for postmenopausal osteoporosis; Report of a WHO Study Group; WHO Technical Report Series 843. Geneva: WHO 1994.

[42] Corless D, Dawson E, Frazer F, Ellis M, Evans SJW, Perry JD, Reisner C, Silver CP, Beer M, Boucher BJ, Cohen RD. Do vitamin D supplements improve the physical capabilities of elderly hospital patients? *Age Ageing* 1985; **14**:76-84.

[43] Chapuy MC, Arlot ME, Delmas PD, Meunier PJ. Effect of calcium and cholecalciferol treatment for three years on hip fractures in elderly women. *BMJ* 1994; **308**:1081-2.

[44] Dawson-Hughes B, Harris SS, Krall EA, Dallal GE. Effect of calcium and vitamin D supplementation on bone density in men and women 65 years of age or older. *N Engl J Med* 1997; **337**:670-6.

[45] Meunier PJ, Chapuy MC, Arlot ME, Delmas PD, Duboeuf F. Can we stop bone loss and prevent hip fractures in the elderly? *Osteoporos Int* 1994; Suppl 1:S71-6.

[46] Cummings SR, Black DM, Nevitt MC, Browner W, Cauley J, Eusrud K, Genant HK, Palermo L, Scott J, Vogt TM. Bone density at various sites for prediction of hip fractures. *Lancet* 1993; **341**:72-5.

[47] Aspray TJ, Francis RM, Prentice A. Evolution of osteoporosis. *Ann Rheum Dis* 1997; **56**:78.

[48] Nakamura T, Turner CH, Yoshikawa T, Slemenda CW, Peacock M, Burr DB, Mizuno Y, Orimo H, Ouchi Y, Johnston CC. Do variations in hip geometry explain differences in hip fracture risk between Japanese and White Americans? *J Bone Min Res* 1994; **9**: 1071-6.

[49] Prentice A. The application of dual-energy X-ray absorptiometry and related techniques to the measurement of bone and body composition. In: PW Davies, TJ Cole (eds):Body Composition Techniques in Health and Disease. Soc Study Hum Biol Symp Series 36. Cambridge: Cambridge University Press, 1995, pp1-13.

[50] Prentice A, Parsons TJ, Cole TJ. Uncritical use of bone mineral density in absorptiometry may lead to size-related artifacts in the identification of bone mineral determinants. *Am J Clin Nutr* 1994; **60**:837-42.

[51] Prentice A, Laskey MA, Shaw J, Cole TJ, Fraser DR. Bone mineral content of Gambian and British children aged 0-36 months. *Bone Miner* 1990; **10**:211-24.

[52] Molgaard C, Thomsen BL, Prentice A, Cole TJ, Michaelsen KF. Whole body bone mineral content in healthy children and adolescents. *Arch Dis Child* 1997; **76**:9-15.

[53] Prentice A, Shaw J, Laskey MA, Cole TJ, Fraser DR. Bone mineral content of British and rural Gambian women aged 18-80+ years. *Bone Miner* 1991; **12**:201-14.

[54] Bhudikanok GS, Wang M-C, Eckert K, Matkin C, Marcus R, Bachrach LK. Differences in bone mineral in young Asian and Caucasian Americans may reflect differences in bone size. *J Bone Min Res* 1996; **11**:1545-56.

[55] Garnero P, Hausherr E, Chapuy MC, Marcelli C, Grandjean H, Muller C, Cormier C, Bréart G, Meunier PJ, Delmas PD. Markers of bone resorption predict hip fracture in elderly women: the EPIDOS prospective study. *J Bone Min Res* 1996; **11**:1531-8.

[56] Department of Health. *Dietary Reference Values for Food Energy and Nutrients for the United Kingdom.* Report on Health and Social Subjects: 41. London: HMSO, 1994.

[57] Commission of the European Communities. *Nutrient and energy intakes for the European Community.* Reports of the Scientific Committee for Food (31st series). Luxembourg: Office for Official Publications of the European Communities, 1993.

[58] Dupin H, Abraham J, Giachetti I. *Apports Nutritionnels Conseillés Pour la Population Française.* 2nd Edition. Paris: TEC and DOC Lavoisier, 1992.

[59] National Health and Medical Research Council. *Recommended Dietary Intakes for use in Australia.* Canberra: Australian Government Publishing Service, 1991.

[60] Nutrition Taskforce (New Zealand). *Food for Health.* Report of the Nutrition Taskforce. Wellington: Department of Health, 1991.

[61] Food and Nutrition Board of the Institute of Medicine. *Dietary Reference Intakes for Calcium, Phosphorus, Magnesium, Vitamin D, and Fluoride.* Washington: National Academy Press, 1997.

[62] Scientific Review Committee. Authority of the Minister of National Health and Welfare. *Nutrition Recommendations.* The Report of the Scientific Review Committee. Canada: Minister of Supply and Services, 1990.

[63] Heaney RP, Weaver CM, Barger-Lux MJ. Food factors influencing calcium availability. *Challenges Mod Med* 1995; **7**:229-41.

[64] Krall EA, Dawson-Hughes B. Relation of fractional ^{47}Ca retention to season and rates of bone loss in healthy postmenopausal women. *J Bone Min Res* 1991; **6**:1323-9.

[65] Weaver CM, Heaney RP, Martin BR, Fitzsimmons ML. Human calcium absorption from whole wheat products. *J Nutr* 1991; **121**:1769-75.

[66] Heaney RP. Nutritional factors in osteoporosis. *Ann Rev Nutr* 1993; **13**:287-316.

[67] The British Nutrition Foundation. *Calcium: The report of the British Nutrition Foundation's Task Force.* London: British Nutrition Foundation, 1989.

[68] Weaver CM, Martin BR, Plawecki KL, Peacock M, Wood OB, Smith DL, Wastney ME. Differences in calcium metabolism between adolescent and adult females. *Am J Clin Nutr* 1995; **61**:577-81.

[69] Fairweather-Tait SJ, Prentice A, Heumann KG, Jarjou LMA, Stirling DM, Wharf SG, Turnlund JR. Effect of calcium supplements and stage of lactation on the efficiency of absorption of calcium by lactating women accustomed to low calcium intakes. *Am J Clin Nutr* 1995; **62**:1188-92.

[70] Malm OJ. Calcium requirement and adaptation in adult men. *Scan J Clin Lab Invest* 1958; **10**(suppl 36).

[71] Whiting SJ, Wood RJ. Adverse effects of high-calcium diets in humans. *Nutr Rev* 1997; **55**:1-9.

[72] Curhan GC, Willett WC, Speizer FE, Spiegelman D, Stampfer MJ. Comparison of dietary calcium with supplemental calcium and other nutrients as factors affecting the risk for kidney stones in women. *Ann Intern Med* 1997; **7**:497-504.

[73] Gleerup A, Rossander-Hulthén L, Gramatkovski E, Hallberg L. Iron absorbtion from the whole diet: comparison of the effect of two different distributions of daily calcium intake. *Am J Clin Nutr* 1995; **61**:97-104.

[74] Prentice A. Maternal calcium requirements during pregnancy and lactation. *Am J Clin Nutr* 1994; **59**:S477-S483.

[75] Prentice A, Dibba B, Jarjou LMA, Laskey MA, Paul AA. Is breast milk calcium concentration influenced by calcium intake during pregnancy? *Lancet* 1994; **344**:411-2.

[76] Kalkwarf HJ, Specker BL, Bianchi DC, Ranz J, Ho M. The effect of calcium supplementation on bone density during lactation and after weaning. *N Engl J Med* 1997; **337**:523-8.

[77] Laskey MA, Jarjou L, Dibba B, Prentice A. Does maternal calcium intake influence the calcium nutrition of the breast-fed baby? *Proc Nutr Soc* 1997; **56**:6A.

[78] Prentice A. Calcium requirements in children. *Nutr Rev* 1995; **53**: 37-40.

[79] Waterlow JC, Schurch B. Causes and mechanisms of linear growth retardation (stunting). *Eur J Clin Nutr* 1994; **48**(suppl 1), S1-S4.

[80] Prentice A, Bates CJ. Adequacy of dietary mineral supply for human bone growth and mineralisation. *Eur J Clin Nutr* 1994; **48**:S161-S177.

[81] Johnston CC, Miller JZ, Slemenda CW, et al. Calcium supplementation and increases in bone mineral density in children. *N Engl J Med* 1992; **327**:82-7.

[82] Lee WTK, Leung SSF, Wang SH, Xu YC, Zeng WP, Lau J, Oppenheimer SJ, Cheng JCY. Double-blind controlled calcium supplementation and bone mineral accretion in children accustomed to a low-calcium diet. *Am J Clin Nutr* 1994; **60**:744-50.

[83] Lee WTK, Leung SSF, Xu YC, Wang SH, Zeng WP, Lau J, Fairweather-Tait SJ. Effects of double-blind controlled calcium supplementation on calcium absorption in Chinese children measured with stable isotopes (^{42}Ca and ^{44}Ca). *Br J Nutr* 1995; **73**:311-21.

[84] Lloyd T, Martel JK, Rollings N, Andon MB, Kulin H, Demers LM, Eggli D, Kieselhorst K, Chinchilli VML. The effect of calcium supplementation and Tanner stage on bone density, content and area in teenage women. *Osteoporos Int* 1996; **6**:276-83.

[85] Bonjour J-P, Carrie A-L, Ferrari S, Claven H, Slosman D, Theintz G, Rizzoli R. Calcium enriched foods and bone mass growth in prepubertal girls: a randomized double-blind, placebo-controlled trial. *J Clin Invest* 1997; **99**:1287-94.

[86] Nowson CA, Green RM, Hopper JL, Sherwin AJ, Young D, Kaymakci B, Guest CS, Smid M, Larkins RG, Wark JD. A co-twin study of the effect of calcium supplementation on bone density during adolescence. *Osteoporos Int* 1997; **7**:219-25.

[87] Dibba B, Prentice A, Poskitt EME, Cole TJ. Calcium supplementation increases the bone mineral status of Gambian children. *Proc Nutr Soc* 1997; **57**:73A.

[88] Slemenda CW, Reister TK, Peacock M, Johnston CC. Bone growth in children following the cessation of calcium supplementation. *J Bone Min Res* 1993; **8**:S154.

[89] Matkovic V, Kostial K, Simonovic I, Buzina R, Brodarec A, Nordin BEC. Bone status and fracture rates in two regions of Yugoslavia. *Am J Clin Nutr* 1979; **32**:540-9.

[90] Soroko S, Holbrook TL, Edelstein S, Barrett-Connor E. Lifetime milk consumption and bone mineral density in older women. *Am J Public Health* 1994; **84**:1319-22.

[91] Kanis JA. Calcium requirements for optimal skeletal health in women. *Calcif Tissue Int* 1991; **49**:S33-41.

[92] Cadogan J, Eastell R, Jones N, Barker M. Milk intake and bone mineral acquisition in adolescent girls: randomised, controlled intervention. *BMJ* 1997; **315**:1255-60.

[93] Chan GM, Hoffman K, McMurray M. The effect of dietary calcium supplementation on pubertal girls' growth and bone mineral status. *J Bone Min Res* 1991; **6**:S240.

[94] Fehily AM, Coles RJ, Evans WD, Elwood PC. Factors affecting bone density in young adults. *Am J Clin Nutr* 1992; **56**:579-86.

[95] Hegsted DM. Calcium and osteoporosis. *J Nutr* 1986; **116**:2316-9.

[96] Slemenda CW, Peacock M, Hui S, Zhou L, Johnston CC. Reduced rates of skeletal remodeling are associated with increased bone mineral density during the development of peak skeletal mass. *J Bone Min Res* 1997; **12**:676-82.

[97] Lee WTK, Leung SSF, Leung DMY, Wang S-H, Xu Y-C, Zeng W-P, Cheng JCY. Bone mineral acquisition in low calcium intake children following the withdrawal of calcium supplement. *Acta Paediatr* 1997; **86**:570-6.

[98] Lee WTK, Leung SSF, Leung DMY, Cheng JCY. A follow-up study on the effects of calcium-supplement withdrawal and puberty on bone acquisition of children. *Am J Clin Nutr* 1996; **64**:71-7.

[99] Lloyd TM, Andon MB, Rollings N, Martel JK, Lanis JR, Demers LM, Eggli DF, Kieselhorst K, Kulin HE. Calcium supplementation and bone mineral density in adolescent girls. *JAMA* 1993; **270**:841-4.

[100] Andon MB, Lloyd T, Matkovic V. Supplementation trials with calcium citrate malate: evidence in favor of increasing the calcium RDA during childhood and adolescence. *J Nutr* 1994; **124**:1412-7S.

[101] Dawson-Hughes B, Dallal GE, Krall EA, Sadowski L, Sahyoun N, Tannenbaum S. A controlled trial of the effect of calcium supplementation on bone density in postmenopausal women. *N Engl J Med* 1990; **323**:878-83.

[102] Ettinger B, Genant HK, Cann CE. Postmenopausal bone loss is prevented by treatment with low-dosage estrogen with calcium. *Ann Intern Med* 1987; **106**:40-5.

[103] Nieves JW, Komar L, Cosman F, Lindsay R. Calcium potentiates the effect of estrogen and calcitonin on bone mass: review and analysis. *Am J Clin Nutr* 1998; **67**:18-24.

[104] Dawson-Hughes B. Osteoporosis treatment and the calcium requirement. *Am J Clin Nutr* 1998; **67**:5-6.

[105] Elders PJM, Lips P, Netelenbos JC, Van Ginkel FC, Khoe E, Van Der Vijgh WJF, Van Der Stelt PF. Long-term effect of calcium supplementation on bone loss in perimenopausal women. *J Bone Min Res* 1994; **9**:963-70.

[106] Aloia JF, Vaswani A, Yeh JK, Ross PL, Flaster E, Dilmanian FA. Calcium supplementation with and without hormone replacement therapy to prevent postmenopausal bone loss. *Ann Intern Med* 1994; **120**:97-103.

[107] Riis B, Thomsen K, Christiansen C. Does calcium supplementation prevent postmenopausal bone loss? *N Engl J Med* 1987; **316**:173-7.

[108] Reid IR, Ames RW, Evans MC, Gamble GD, Sharpe SJ. Long-term effects of calcium supplementation on bone loss and fractures in postmenopausal women: a randomised controlled trial. *Am J Med* 1995; **98**:331-5.

[109] Reid IR, Ames RW, Evans MC, Gamble GD, Sharpe SJ. Effect of calcium supplementation on bone loss in postmenopausal women. *N Engl J Med* 1993; **328**:460-4.

[110] Prince RP, Devine A, Dick I, Criddle A, Kerr D, Kent N, Price R, Randell A. The effects of calcium supplementation (milk powder or tablets) and exercise on bone density in postmenopausal women. *J Bone Min Res* 1995; **10**:1068-75.

[111] Recker R, Hinders S, Davies KM, Heaney RP, Stegman MR, Lappe JM, Kimmel DB. Correcting calcium nutritional deficiency prevents spine fractures in elderly women. *J Bone Min Res* 1996; **11**:1961-6.

[112] Chevalley T, Rizzoli R, Nydegger V, Slosman D, Rapin C-H, Michel J, Vasey J, Bonjour J-P. Effects of calcium supplements on femoral bone mineral density and vertebral fracture rate in vitamin-D replete elderly patients. *Osteoporos Int* 1994; **4**:245-52.

[113] Lau EMC, Woo J, Leung PC, Swaminathan R, Leung D. The effects of calcium supplementation and exercise on bone density in elderly Chinese women. *Osteoporos Int* 1992; **2**:168-73.

[114] Riggs BL, O'Fallon WM, Muhs J, O'Connor MK, Kumar R, Melton III LJ. Long-term effects of calcium supplementation on serum parathyroid hormone level, bone turnover, and bone loss in elderly women. *J Bone Min Res* 1998; **13**:168-74.

[115] Smith EL, Gilligan C, Smith PE, Sempos CT. Calcium supplementation and bone loss in middle-aged women. *Am J Clin Nutr* 1989; **50**:833-42.

[116] Hansson T, Roo B. The effect of fluoride and calcium on spinal bone mineral content: a controlled, prospective (3 years) study. *Calcif Tissue Int* 1987; **40**:315-7.

[117] Polley KJ, Nordin BEC, Baghurst PA, Walker CJ. Effect of calcium supplementation on forearm bone mineral content in postmenopausal women: a prospective sequential controlled trial. *J Nutr* 1987; **117**:1929-35.

[118] Horsman A, Gallagher JC, Simpson M, Nordin BEC. Prospective trial of oestrogen and calcium in post-menopausal women. *BMJ* 1977; **ii**:789-92.

[119] Recker RR, Saville PD, Heavey RP. Effect of estrogens and calcium carbonate on bone loss in postmenopausal women. *Ann Intern Med* 1977; **87**:649-55.

[120] Nordin BEC, Horsman A, Crilly RG, Marshall DH, Simpson M. Treatment of spinal osteoporosis in postmenopausal women. *BMJ* 1980; **280**:451-5.

[121] Lamke B, Sjobergh E, Sylven M. Bone mineral content in women with Colles fracture: effect of calcium supplementation. *Acta Orthop Scand* 1978; **49**:143-9.

[122] Cooper C, Barker DJ, Wickham C. Physical activity, muscle strength, and calcium intake in fracture of the proximal femur in Britain. *BMJ* 1988; **297**:1443-6.

[123] Cumming RG, Klineberg R. Case-control study of risk factors for hip fractures in the elderly. *Am J Epidemiol* 1994; **139**:493-503.

[124] Kreiger N, Gross A, Hunter G. Dietary factors and fracture in postmenopausal women: a case-control study. *Int J Epidemiol* 1992; **21**:953-8.

[125] Lau E, Donnan S, Barker DJ, Cooper C. Physical activity and calcium intake in fracture of the proximal femur in Hong Kong. *BMJ* 1988; **297**:1441-3.

[126] Johnell OF, Gullberg B, Kanis JA, Allander E, Elffors L, Dequeker J, Dilsen G, Genarri C, Lopes Vaz A, Lyritis G, Mazzuoli G, Miravet L, Passeri M, Cano RP, Rapado A, Ribot C. Risk factors for hip fracture in European women: the MEDOS Study. *J Bone Min Res* 1995; **10**:1802-15.

[127] Wickham CAC, Walsh K, Cooper C, Barker DJP, Margetts BM, Morris J, Bruce SA. Dietary calcium, physical activity, and risk of hip fracture: a prospective study. *BMJ* 1989; **299**:889-92.

[128] Cummings SR, Nevitt MC, Browner WS, Stone K, Fox KM, Ensrud KE, Cauley J, Black D, Vogt TM. Risk factors for hip fractures in white women. *N Engl J Med* 1995; **332**:767-73.

[129] Holbrook TL, Barrett-Connor E, Wingard DL. Dietary calcium and risk of hip fracture: 14 year prospective population study. *Lancet* 1988; **ii**:1046-9.

[130] Cumming RG, Nevitt MC. Calcium for prevention of osteoporotic fractures in postmenopausal women. *J Bone Min Res* 1997; **12**:1321-9.

[131] De Laet CEDH, van Hout BA, Burger H, Hofman A, Pols HAP. Bone density and risk of hip fracture in men and women: cross sectional analysis. *BMJ* 1997; **315**:221-5.

[132] Slemenda CW, Christian CC, Reed T, Reister TK, Williams CJ, Johnston CC Jr. Long-term bone loss in men: effects of genetic and environmental factors. *Ann Intern Med* 1992; **117**:286-91.

[133] Chapuy MC, Arlot ME, Duboeuf F, Brun J, Crouzet B, Arnaud MS, Delmas PD, Meunier PJ. Vitamin D_3 and calcium to prevent hip fractures in elderly women. *N Engl J Med* 1992; **327**:1637-42.

[134] Orwoll ES, Oviatt SK, McClung MR, Deftos LJ, Sexton G. The rate of bone mineral loss in normal men and the effects of calcium and cholecalciferol supplementation. *Ann Intern Med* 1990; **112**:29-34.

[135] Laskey MA, Prentice A, Hanratty LA, Jarjou LMA, Dibba B, Beavan S, Cole TJ. Bone changes after 3 months of lactation: influence of calcium intake, breast-milk output and vitamin-D receptor genotype. *Am J Clin Nutr* 1998; **67**:685-92.

[136] Sowers MF. Pregnancy and lactation as risk factors for subsequent bone loss and osteoporosis. *J Bone Min Res* 1996; **11**:1052-60.

[137] Prentice A. Calcium supplementation during breast-feeding. *N Engl J Med* 1997; **337**:558-9.

[138] Laskey MA, Prentice A. Longitudinal bone mineral changes during lactation and after weaning. *Osteoporos Int* (in press).

[139] Laskey MA, Prentice A. Effect of pregnancy on recovery of lactational bone loss. *Lancet* 1997; **349**:1518-9.

[140] Lopez JM, Gonzalez G, Reyes V, Campino C, Diaz S. Bone turnover and density in healthy women during breastfeeding and after weaning. *Osteoporos Int* 1996; **6**:153-9.

[141] Hayslip CC, Klein TA, Wray HL, Duncan WE. The effects of lactation on bone mineral content in healthy postpartum women. *Obstet Gynecol* 1989; **73**:588-92.

[142] Sowers MF, Corton G, Shapiro B, Jannausch ML, Crutchfield M, Smith ML, Randolph JF, Hollis B. Changes in bone density with lactation. *JAMA* 1993; **269**:3130-5.

[143] Krebs NF, Reidinger CJ, Robertson AD, Brenner M. Bone mineral density changes during lactation: maternal, dietary and biochemical correlates. *Am J Clin Nutr* 1997; **65**:1738-46.

[144] Kent GN, Price RI, Gutteridge DH, May KD, Allen JR, Smith M, Evans DV, Bhagat CI. Site-specific reduction in bone loss by calcium supplements in normal lactation. *Osteoporos Int* 1995; **5**:315.

[145] Prentice A, Jarjou LMA, Cole TJ, Stirling DM, Dibba B, Fairweather-Tait S. Calcium requirements of lactating Gambian mothers: effects of a calcium supplement on breast-milk calcium concentration, maternal bone mineral content, and urinary calcium excretion. *Am J Clin Nutr 1995*; **62**:58-67.

[146] Cross NA, Hillman LS, Allen SH, Krause GF. Changes in bone mineral density and markers of bone remodeling during lactation and postweaning in women consuming high amounts of calcium. *J Bone Min Res* 1995; **10**:1312-20.

[147] Reichel H, Koeffler HP, Norman AW. The role of the vitamin D endocrine system in health and disease. *N Engl J Med* 1989; **320**:980-91.

[148] Price PA, Baukol SA. 1,25-dihydroxyvitamin D_3 increases synthesis of the vitamin K-dependent bone protein by osteosarcoma cells. *J Biol Chem* 1980; **255**:11660-3.

[149] Gloth FM III, Grundberg CM, Hollis BW, Haddad JG, Tobin JD. Vitamin D deficiency in homebound elderly persons. *JAMA* 1995; **274**:1683-6.

[150] Utiger RD. The need for more vitamin D. *N Engl J Med* 1998; **338**:828-9.

[151] Guillemant J, Guillemant S. Acute PTH response to oral calcium load and seasonal variation of vitamin D status in healthy young adult subjects. *Eur J Clin Nutr* 1996; **50**:469-72.

[152] Lips P, Wiersinga A, van Ginkel FC, Jongen MJM, Netelenbos JC, Hackeng WHL, Delmas PD, van der Vijgn WJF. The effect of vitamin D supplementation on vitamin D status and parathyroid function in elderly subjects. *J Clin Endocrinol Metab* 1988; **67**:644-50.

[153] Sherman SS, Hollis BW, Tobin JD. Vitamin D status and related parameters in a healthy population: the effects of age, sex, and season. *J Clin Endocrinol Metab* 1990; **71**:405-13.

[154] Khaw KT, Sneyd MJ, Compston J. Bone density, parathyroid hormone and 25-hydroxyvitamin D concentrations in middle aged women. *BMJ* 1992; **350**: 263-7.

[155] Hegarty V, Woodhouse P, Khaw KT. Seasonal variation in parathyroid hormone and vitamin D concentrations in an elderly population. *Age Ageing* 1994; **23**:478-82.

[156] Landin-Wilhelmsen K, Wilhelmsen L, Wilske J, Lappas G, Rosén T, Lindstedt G, Lundberg P-A, Bengtsson B-A. Sunlight increases serum 25(OH)vitamin D concentration whereas $1,25(OH)_2D_3$ is unaffected. Results from a general population study in Göteborg, Sweden (The WHO MONICA Project). *Eur J Clin Nutr* 1995; **49**:400-7.

[157] Kinyamu HK, Gallagher JC, Rafferty KA, Balhorn KE. Dietary calcium and vitamin D intake in elderly women: effect on serum parathyroid hormone and vitamin D metabolites. *Am J Clin Nutr* 1998; **67**:342-8.

[158] Malabanan A, Veronikis IE, Holick MF. Redefining vitamin D insufficiency. *Lancet* 1998; **351**:805-6.

[159] Solanki T, Hyatt RH, Kemm JR, Hughes EA, Cowan RA. Are elderly Asians in Britain at a high risk of vitamin D deficiency and osteomalacia? *Age Ageing* 1995; **24**:103-7.

[160] Ooms ME, Roos JC, Bezemer PD, Van der Vijch WJF, Bouter LM, Lips P. Prevention of bone loss by vitamin D supplementation in elderly women: a randomised double blind trial. *J Clin Endocrinol Metab* 1995; **80**:1052-8.

[161] Chapuy MC, Preziosi P, Maamer M, Arnaud S, Galan P, Hercberg S, Meunier PJ. Prevalence of vitamin D insufficiency in an adult population. *Osteoporos Int* 1997; **7**:439-43.

[162] Dawson-Hughes B, Harris SS, Dallal GE. Plasma calcidiol, season, and serum parathyroid hormone concentrations in healthy elderly men and women. *Am J Clin Nutr* 1997; **65**:67-71.

[163] Krall EA, Sahyoun N, Tannenbaum S, Dallal GE, Dawson-Hughes B. Effect of vitamin D intake on seasonal variations in parathyroid hormone secretion in postmenopausal women. *N Engl J Med* 1989; **321**:1777-83.

[164] Stamp TCB, Round JM. Seasonal changes in human plasma levels of 25(OH)vitamin D. *Nature* 1974; **247**:563-5.

[165] McLaughlin M, Fairney A, Lester E, Raggatt RP, Brown DJ, Will MR. Seasonal variations in serum 25-hydroxycholecalciferol in healthy people. *Lancet* 1974; **i**:536-7.

[166] Lawson DEM, Paul AA, Black AE, Cole TJ, Mandal AR, Davie M. Relative contributions of diet and sunlight to vitamin D state in the elderly. *BMJ* 1979; **2**:303-8.

[167] McKenna MJ. Differences in vitamin D status between countries in young adults and the elderly. *Am J Clin Nutr* 1992; **93**:69-77.

[168] Prentice A, Yan L, Landing MAJ, Dibba B, Laskey A, Stirling DH, Fairweather-Tait S. Vitamin D status does not influence the breast-milk calcium concentration of lactating mothers accustomed to a low calcium intake. *Acta Paediatr* 1997; **86**:1006-8.

[169] Dawson-Hughes B, Dallas GE, Krall EA, Harris S, Sokoll LJ, Fakoner C. Effect of vitamin D supplementation in wintertime and overall bone loss in healthy postmenopausal women. *Ann Intern Med* 1991; **115**:505-12.

[170] Davies M, Mawer EB, Hann JT, Stephens WP, Taylor JL. Vitamin D prophylaxis in the elderly: a simple effective method suitable for large populations. *Age Ageing* 1985; **14**:349-54.

[171] Grimley Evans J. The epidemiology of osteoporosis. *Rev Clin Gerontol* 1993; **3**:13-29.

[172] Jacobsen SJ, Goldberg J, Miles TP, Brody JA, Stiers W, Rimm AA. Seasonal variation in the incidence of hip fracture among white persons aged 65 years and older in the United States. *Am J Epidemiol* 1991; **133**:996-1004.

[173] MacLaughlin J, Holick MF. Aging decreases the capacity of human skin to produce vitamin D_3. *J Clin Invest* 1985; **76**:1536-8.

[174] Holick MF, Matsuoka LY, Wortsman J. Age, vitamin D and solar ultraviolet [letter]. *Lancet* 1989; **2**:1104-5.

[175] Barragry JM, France MW, Corless D, Gupta SP, Switala S, Boucher BJ, Cohen RD. Intestinal cholecalciferol absorption in the elderly and in younger adults. *Clin Sci Mol Med* 1978; **55**:213-20.

[176] Tsai K-S, Heath III H, Kumar R, Riggs BL. Impaired vitamin D metabolism with ageing in women. *J Clin Invest* 1984; **73**:1668-72.

[177] Clemens TL, Adams JS, Henderson SL, Holick MF. Increased skin pigment reduces the capacity of skin to synthesise vitamin D_3. *Lancet* 1982; **1**:74-6.

[178] Finch PJ, Ang L, Colston KW, Nisbet J, Maxwell JD. Blunted seasonal variation in serum 25-hydroxyvitamin D and increased risk of osteomalacia in vegetarian London Asians. *Eur J Clin Nutr* 1992; **42**:509-15.

[179] Matsuoka LY, Wortsman J, Daumenberg MJ, Hollis BW, Lu Z, Holick MF. Clothing prevents ultraviolet-B radiation-dependent photosynthesis of vitamin D_3. *J Clin Endocrinol Metab* 1992; **75**:1099-103.

[180] Henderson FB, Dunnigan MG, McIntosh WB, Abdul-Motaal A, Hole D. Asian osteomalacia is determined by dietary factors when exposure to ultra-violet radiation is restricted: a risk factor model. *Q J Med* 1990; **76**: 923-33.

[181] Blank S, Scanlon KS, Sinks TH, Lett S, Falk H. An outbreak of hypervitaminosis D associated with the overfortification of milk from a home-delivery dairy. *Am J Public Health* 1995; **85**:656-9.

[182] Byrne PM, Freaney R, McKenna MJ. Vitamin D supplementation in the elderly: review of safety and effectiveness of different regimes. *Calcif Tissue Int* 1995; **56**:518-20.

[183] National Radiation Protection Board. *Board Statement on Effects of Ultraviolet Radiation on Human Health*. Didcot: National Radiation Protection Board, 1995.

[184] Department of Health. *The Nutrition of Elderly People*. Report on Health and Social Subjects:43. London: HMSO, 1992.

[185] Brooke OG, Brown IRF, Bone CDM, Carter ND, Cleeve HJW, Maxwell JD, Robinson VP, Winder SM. Vitamin D supplements in pregnant Asian women: effects on calcium status and fetal growth. *BMJ* 1980; **280**:751-4.

[186] Specker BL, Vierra NE, O'Brien KO, Ho ML, Heubi JE, Abrams SA, Yergey AL. Calcium kinetics in lactating women with low and high calcium intakes. *Am J Clin Nutr* 1994; **59**:593-9.

[187] Mawer EB, Stanbury SW, Robinson MJ, James J, Close C. Vitamin D nutrition and vitamin D metabolism in the premature human neonate. *Clin Endocrinol* 1986; **25**:641-9.

[188] Department of Health. *Weaning and the Weaning Diet*. Report on Health and Social Subjects: 45. London: HMSO, 1994.

[189] Henderson FB, Dunnigan MG, McIntosh WB, Abdul-Motaal A, Gettinby G, Glekin BM. The importance of limited exposure to ultra-violet radiation and dietary factors in the aetiology of Asian rickets: a risk factor model. *Q J Med* 1987; **63**: 413-25.

[190] El-Sonbaty MR, Abdul-Ghaffar NU. Vitamin D deficiency in veiled Kuwaiti women. *Eur J Clin Nutr* 1996; **50**:315-8.

[191] Colhoun H, Prescott-Clarke P. Health Survey for England 1994. London: HMSO, 1996.

[192] Baker MR, McDonnell H, Peacock M, Nordin BEC. Plasma 25-hydroxy vitamin D concentrations in patients with fractures of the femoral neck. *BMJ* 1979; **1**:589.

[193] Aaron JE, Gallagher JC, Anderson J, Stasiak L, Longton EB, Nordin BEC, Nicholson M. Frequency of osteomalacia in fractures of the proximal femur. *Lancet* 1974; **i**:229-33.

[194] Compston JR, Vedi S, Croucher PI. Low prevalence of osteomalacia in elderly patients with hip fracture. *Age Ageing* 1991; **20**:132-4.

[195] Hordon LD, Peacock M. Osteomalacia and osteoporosis in femoral neck fracture. *Bone Miner* 1990; **11**: 247-59.

[196] Riggs L, Melton LJ. Evidence for two distinct syndromes of involutional osteoporosis. *Am J Med* 1983; **75**:899-901.

[197] Christiansen C, Christensen MS, McNair P, Hagen C, Stocklund KE, Transbol I. Prevention of early bone loss: controlled 2-year study in 315 normal females. *Eur J Clin Invest* 1980; **10**:273-9.

[198] Lips P, Graafmans WC, Ooms ME, Bezemer D, Bouter LM. Vitamin D supplementation and fracture incidence in elderly persons. A randomized, placebo-controlled clinical trial. *Ann Intern Med* 1996; **124**:400-6.

[199] Heikinheimo RJ, Inkovaara JA, Harju EJ, Haavisto MV, Kaarela RH, Kataja JM, Kokko AM, Kolho LA, Rajala SA. Annual injection of vitamin D and fractures of aged bones. *Calcif Tissue Int* 1992; **51**:105-110.

[200] Flicker L, Hopper JL, Rodgers L, Kaymakci B, Green RW, Wark JD. Bone density in elderly women: a twin study. *J Bone Min Res* 1995; **10**:1607-13.

[201] Sykes B. Bone disease cracks genetics. *Nature* 1990; **348**:18-20.

[202] Grant SFA, Reid DM, Blake G, Herd R, Fogelman I, Ralston SH. Reduced bone density and osteoporosis associated with a polymorphic Sp1 binding site in the collagen type 1∞1 gene. *Nat Genet* 1996; **14**:203-5.

[203] Kobayashi S, Inoue S, Hosoi T, Ouchi Y, Shiraki M, Orimo H. Association of bone mineral density with polymorphism of the estrogen receptor gene. *J Bone Min Res* 1996; **11**:306-11.

[204] Eisman JA. Vitamin D receptor gene alleles and osteoporosis: an affirmative view. *J Bone Min Res* 1995; **10**:1289-93.

[205] Peacock M. Vitamin D receptor gene alleles and osteoporosis: a contrasting view. *J Bone Min Res* 1995; **10**:1294-7.

[206] Cooper GS, Umbach DM. Are vitamin D receptor polymorphisms associated with bone mineral density? A meta-analysis. *J Bone Min Res* 1996; **11**:1841-9.

[207] Krall EA, Parry P, Lichter JB, Dawson-Hughes B. Vitamin D receptor alleles and rates of bone loss: influence of years since menopause and calcium intake. *J Bone Min Res* 1995; **10**:978-84.

[208] Dawson-Hughes B, Harris SS, Finnerman S. Calcium absorption on high and low calcium intakes in relation to vitamin D receptor genotype. *J Clin Endocrinol Metab* 1995; **80**:3657-61.

[209] Baumgartner RN, Stauber PM, Koehler KM, Romero L, Garry PJ. Associations of fat and muscle masses with bone mineral in elderly men and women. *Am J Clin Nutr* 1996; **63**:365-72.

[210] Parsons TJ, van Dusseldorp M, van Vliet M, van de Werken K, Schaafsma G, van Staveren WA. Reduced bone mass in Dutch adolescents fed macrobiotic diet in early life. *J Bone Min Res* 1997; **12**:1486-94.

[211] Salisbury JJ, Mitchell JE. Bone mineral density and anorexia nervosa in women. *Am J Psychiatry* 1991; **48**:768-74.

[212] Prentice A. Is nutrition important in osteoporosis? *Proc Nut Soc* 1997; **56**:357-67.

[213] Delmi M, Rapin C-H, Bengoa J-M, Delmas PD, Vasey H, Bonjour J-P. Dietary supplementation in elderly patients with fractured neck of femur. *Lancet* 1990; **335**:1013-6.

[214] Abelow BJ, Holford TR, Insogna KL. Cross-cultural association between dietary animal protein and hip fracture; a hypothesis. *Calcif Tissue Int* 1992; **50**:14-18.

[215] Feskanich D, Willett WC, Stampfer MJ, Colditz GA. Protein consumption and bone fractures in women. *Am J Epidemiol* 1996; **143**:472-9.

[216] Metz JA, Anderson JJB, Gallagher PN. Intakes of calcium, phosphorus and protein and physical activity level are related to radial bone mass in young adult women. *Am J Clin Nutr* 1993; **58**:537-42.

[217] Hernández-Avila M, Stampfer MJ, Ravnikar VA, Willett WC, Schiff I, Francis M, Longscope C, McKinlay SM. Caffeine and other predictors of bone density among pre- and perimenopausal women. *Epidemiology* 1993; **4**:129-34.

[218] Binkley NC, Suttie JW. Vitamin K nutrition and osteoporosis. *J Nutr* 1995; **125**:1812-21.

[219] Shearer MJ. The roles of vitamins D and K in bone health and osteoporosis prevention. *Proc Nutr Soc* 1997; **56**:915-37.

[220] Sokoll LJ, Booth SL, O'Brien ME, Davidson KW, Tsaioun KI, Sadowski JA. Changes in serum osteocalcin, plasma phylloquinone, and urinary γ-carboxyglutamic acid in response to altered intakes of dietary phylloquinone in human subjects. *Am J Clin Nutr* 1997; **65**:779-84.

[221] Szulc P, Chapuy MC, Meunier PJ, Delmas PD. Serum undercarboxylated osteocalcin is a marker of the risk of hip fracture in elderly women. *J Clin Invest* 1993; **91**:1769-74.

[222] Vergnaud P, Garnero P, Meunier PJ, Breart G, Kamihagi K, Delmas PD. Undercarboxylated osteocalcin measured with specific immunoassay predicts hip fracture in elderly women: the EPIDOS study. *J Clin Endocrinol Metab* 1997; **82**:717-8.

[223] Szulc P, Arlot M, Chapuy M-C, Duboeuf F, Meunier PJ, Delmas PD. Serum undercarboxylated osteocalcin correlates with hip bone mineral density in elderly women. *J Bone Min Res* 1994; **9**:1591-5.

[224] Gunnes M, Lehmann EH. Dietary calcium, saturated fat, fiber and vitamin C as predictors of forearm cortical and trabecular bone-mineral density in healthy children and adolescents. *Acta Paediatr* 1995; **84**:388-92.

[225] New SA, Bolton-Smith C, Grubb DA, Reid DM. Nutritional influences on bone mineral density: a cross-sectional study in premenopausal women. *Am J Clin Nutr* 1997; **65**:1831-9.

[226] Leveille SG, LaCroix AZ, Keopsell TD, Beresford SA, Van Belle G, Buchner DM. Dietary vitamin C and bone mineral density in postmenopausal women in Washington State, USA. *J Epidemiol Community Health* 1997; **51**:479-85.

[227] Reginster JY, Strause LG, Saltman P, Franchimont P. Trace elements and postmenopausal osteoporosis: a preliminary study of decreased serum manganese. *Med Sci Res* 1988; **16**:337-8.

[228] Massey LK, Whiting SJ. Dietary salt, urinary calcium, and bone loss. *J Bone Min Res* 1996; **6**:731-6.

[229] Shortt C, Madden A, Flynn A, Morrissey PA. Influence of dietary sodium intake on urinary calcium excretion in selected Irish individuals. *Eur J Clin Nutr* 1988; **42**:595-603.

[230] Matkovic V, Ilich JZ, Andon MB, Hsieh LC, Tzagournis MA, Lagger BJ, Goel PK. Urinary calcium, sodium and bone mass of young females. *Am J Clin Nutr* 1995; **62**:417-25.

[231] Devine A, Criddle RA, Dick IM, Kerr DA, Prince RL. A longitudinal study of the effect of sodium and calcium intakes on regional bone density in postmenopausal women. *Am J Clin Nutr* 1995; **62**:740-5.

[232] Dawson-Hughes B, Fowler SE, Dalsky G, Gallagher C. Sodium excretion influences calcium homeostasis in elderly men and women. *J Nutr* 1996; **126**:2107-12.

[233] New SA, Tredger JA, Smith R, Greenacre MC, Grubb DA, Reid DM. Association between present dietary intake and bone health in postmenopausal and elderly Scottish women. *Proc Nutr Soc* 1998;**57**:(in press).

[234] Department of Health. *Nutritional Aspects of Cardiovascular Disease*. Report on Health and Social Subjects: 46. London: HMSO, 1994.

[235] Health Education Authority. *Eight Guidelines for a Healthy Diet: a Guide for Nutrition Educators*. London: Health Education Authority, 1997.

[236] Kleerekoper M, Balena R. Fluorides and osteoporosis. *Ann Rev Nutr* 1991; **11**:309-24.

[237] Beattie JH, Avenell A. Trace element nutrition and bone metabolism. *Nutr Res Rev* 1992; **5**:167-88.

[238] Gordon SL, Corbin SB. Summary of Workshop on Drinking Water Fluoride Influence on Hip Fracture on Bone Health. *Osteoporos Int* 1992; **2**:109-17.

[239] Hillier S, Inship H, Coggon D, Cooper C. Water fluoridation and osteoporotic fracture. *Community Dent Health* 1996; **13**(suppl 2):63-8.

[240] Pak CYC, Zerwekh JE, Antich P. Anabolic effects of fluoride on bone. *Tr Endocrin Metab* 1995; **6**:229-34.

[241] Higashi A, Nakamura T, Nishiyama S, Matsukara M, Tomoeda S, Futagoishi Y, Shinohara M, Matsuda I. Zinc kinetics in patients with bone demineralization due to physical immobilization. *J Am Coll Nutr* 1993; **12**:61-5.

[242] Ninh NX, Thissen JP, Collette L, Gerard G, Khoi HH, Ketelslegers JM. Zinc supplementation increases growth and circulating insulin-like growth factor 1 (IGF-1) in growth-retarded Vietnamese children. *Am J Clin Nutr* 1996; **63**:514-9.

[243] Eaton-Evans J, McIlrath EM, Jackson WE, McCartney H, Strain JJ. Copper supplementation and the maintenance of bone mineral density in middle-aged women. *J Trace Elem Exp Med* 1996; **9**:87-94.

[244] Freudenheim JL, Johnson NE, Smith EL. Relationship between usual nutrient intake and bone mineral content of women 35-65 years of age: longitudinal and cross-sectional analysis. *Am J Clin Nutr* 1986; **44**:863-76.

[245] Reynolds TM, Marshall PD, Brain AM. Hip fracture patients may be vitamin B6 deficient: controlled study of serum pyridoxal-5-phosphate. *Acta Orthop Scand* 1992; **63**:635-8.

[246] Meacham SL, Taper LJ, Volpe SL. Effects of boron supplementation on bone mineral density and dietary, blood, and urinary calcium, phosphorus, magnesium and boron in female athletes. *Environ Health Perspect* 1994; **102**:79-82.

[247] Reid DM, New SA. Nutritional influence on bone mass. *Proc Nutr Soc* 1997; **56**:977-87.

[248] Mason KE. A conspectus of research on copper metabolism and requirements of man. *J Nutr* 1979; **109**:1979-2066.

[249] Strause L, Saltman P, Smith KT, Bracker M, Andon MB. Spinal bone loss in postmenopausal women supplemented with calcium and trace minerals. *J Nutr* 1994; **124**:1060-4.

[250] Tesar R, Notelovitz M, Shim E, Kauwell G, Brown J. Axial and peripheral bone density and nutrient intakes of postmenopausal vegetarian and omnivorous women. *Am J Clin Nutr* 1992; **56**:699-704.

[251] Lloyd T, Schaeffer JM, Walker MA, Demers LM. Urinary hormonal concentrations and spinal bone densities of premenopausal vegetarian and non-vegetarian women. *Am J Clin Nutr* 1991; **54**:1005-10.

[252] Chiu JF, Lan SJ, Yang CY, Yao WJ, Su LH, Hsieh CC. Long-term vegetarian diet and bone mineral density in postmenopausal Taiwanese women. *Calcif Tissue Int* 1997; **60**:245-9.

[253] Felson DT, Kiel DP, Anderson JJ, Kannel WB. Alcohol consumption and hip fractures: the Framingham study. *Am J Epidemiol* 1988; **128**:1102-10.

[254] Eaton-Evans J, McIlrath EM, Jackson WE, Bradley P, Strain JJ. Dietary factors and vertebral bone density in perimenopausal women from a general medical practice in Northern Ireland. *Proc Nutr Soc* 1993; **52**:44A.

[255] Barrett-Connor E, Chang JC, Edelstein SL. Coffee-associated osteoporosis offset by daily milk consumption. *JAMA* 1994; **271**(4):280-3.

[256] Harris SS, Dawson-Hughes B. Caffeine and bone loss in healthy postmenopausal women. *Am J Clin Nutr* 1994; **60**:573-8.

[257] Lloyd T, Rollings N, Eggli DF, Kieselhorst K, Chinchilli VM. Dietary caffeine intake and bone status of postmenopausal women. *Am J Clin Nutr* 1997; **65**:1826-30.

[258] Kuiper GG, Carlsson B, Grandien K, Enmark E, Haggblad J, Nilsson S, Gustafsson JA. Comparison of the ligand binding specificity and transcript tissue distribution of estrogen receptors alpha and beta. *Endocrinology* 1997; **138**:863-70.

[259] Brandi ML. Natural and synthetic isoflavones in the prevention and treatment of chronic diseases. *Calcif Tissue Int* 1997; **60**(suppl 1):S5-S8.

[260] Purdie DW. Bone mineral metabolism and reproduction. *Contemp Rev Obstet Gynecol* 1989; **1**:214-21.

[261] Falch JA, Sandvik L. Perimenopausal appendicular bone loss: a 10 year prospective study. *Bone* 1990; **11**:425-8.

[262] Manolagas SC, Jilka RL. Bone marrow cytokines and bone remodelling. *N Engl J Med* 1995; **332**:305-11.

[263] Grimley Evans J. Incidence of proximal femoral fracture. *Lancet* 1985; **i**:925-6.

[264] Editorial. Anti-oestrogenic effect of cigarette smoking. *Lancet* 1986; **ii**:1433.

[265] Kiel DP, Baron JA, Anderson JJ, Hannan MT, Felson DT. Smoking eliminates the protective effect of oral estrogens on the risk for hip fracture among women. *Ann Intern Med* 1992; **116**:716-21.

[266] Law MR, Hackshaw AK. A meta-analysis of cigarette smoking, bone mineral density and risk of hip fracture: recognition of a major effect. *BMJ* 1997; **315**:841-6.

[267] Torgerson DJ, Reid DM, Campbell MK. Meta-analysis of cigarette smoking, bone mineral density, and risk of hip fracture. *BMJ* 1998; **316**:1017.

[268] Cooper C, Wickham C, Coggon D. Sedentary work in middle life and fracture of the proximal femur. *Br J Ind Med* 1990; **47**:69-70.

[269] Jaglal SB, Kreiger N, Darlington G. Past and recent physical activity and risk of hip fracture. *Am J Epidemiol* 1993; **138**:107-118.

[270] Frost H. Suggested fundamental concepts in skeletal physiology. *Calcif Tissue Int* 1993; **52**:1-4.

[271] Taaffe DR, Robinson TL, Snow CM, Marcus R. High impact exercise promotes bone gain in well-trained female athletes. *J Bone Min Res* 1997; **12**:255-60.

[272] Bassey EJ, Ramsdale SJ. Increase in femoral bone density in young women following high impact exercise. *Osteoporos Int* 1994; **4**:72-5.

[273] Chow RK, Harrison JE, Notarius C. Effect of two randomised exercise programmes on bone mass of healthy postmenopausal women. *BMJ* 1987; **295**:1441-4.

[274] Ayalon J, Simkin A, Leichter I, Raifmann S. Dynamic bone loading exercises for postmenopausal women: effect on the density of the distal radius. *Arch Phys Med Rehabil* 1987; **68**:280-3.

[275] Dalsky G. Weight-bearing exercise training and lumbar bone mineral content in postmenopausal women. *Ann Intern Med* 1988; **108**:824-8.

[276] Kohrt W, Snead D, Slatopolsky E, Birge SJ. Additive effects of weight-bearing exercise and estrogen on bone mineral density in older women. *J Bone Min Res* 1995; **10**:1303-11.

[277] Krall EA, Dawson-Hughes B. Walking is related to bone density and rates of loss. *Am J Med* 1994; **96**:20-26.

[278] Grimston SK, Willows ND, Hanley DA. Mechanical loading regime and its relation to bone mineral density in children. *Med Sci Sports Exerc* 1993; **25**:1203-13.

[279] Rico H, Revilla M, Hernandez ER, Gomez-Castresana F, Villa LF. Bone mineral content and body composition in postpubertal cyclist boys. *Bone* 1993; **14**:93-5.

[280] Nelson ME, Fiatarone MA, Morganti CM, Trice I, Greenberg RA, Evans WJ. Effects of high-intensity strength training on multiple risk factors for osteoporotic fractures. *JAMA* 1994; **272**:1909-14.

[281] Kerr D, Morton A, Dick I, Prince R. Exercise effects on bone mass are site-specific and load dependent. *J Bone Min Res* 1996; **11**:218-25.

[282] Sinaki M, Wahner HW, Offord KP, Hodgson SF. Efficacy of nonloading exercises in prevention of vertebral bone loss in postmenopausal women: a controlled trial. *Mayo Clin Proc* 1989; **64**:762-9.

[283] McCartney N, Hicks AL, Martin J, Webber CE. Long-term resistance training in the elderly: effects on dynamic strength, exercise capacity, muscle and bone. *J Gerontol* Series A 1995; **50**:B97-104.

[284] Department of Health. *More People, More Activity, More Often*. London: Department of Health, 1995.

[285] Ministry of Agriculture, Fisheries and Food. *National Food Survey*. Annual reports of the National Food Survey Committee. London: HMSO/The Stationery Office, 1949-1997.

[286] Gregory J, Foster K, Tyler HA, Wiseman M. *The dietary and nutritional survey of British adults*. London: HMSO, 1990.

[287] Gregory J, Collins DL, Davies PSW, Hughes JM, Clarke PC. *National Diet and Nutrition Survey: Children aged 1½ to 4½ years: Volume 1: Report of the diet and nutrition survey*. London: HMSO, 1995.

[288] Finch S, Doyle W, Lowe C, Bates CJ, Prentice A, Smithers G, Clarke PC. *National Diet and Nutrition Survey: people aged 65 years and over. Volume 1: Report of the diet and nutrition survey*. London: The Stationery Office, 1998.

[289] Department of Health and Social Security. *A Nutrition survey of Pre-School Children 1967-1968*. Report on Health and Social Subjects: 10. London: HMSO, 1975.

[290] Department of Health and Social Security. *Nutrition and Health in Old Age*. Report on Health and Social Subjects: 16. London: HMSO, 1979.

[291] Couzy F, Kastenmayer P, Vigo M, Clough J, Minoz-Box R, Barclay DV. Calcium bioavailability from a calcium- and sulfate-rich mineral water, compared with milk, in young adult women. *Am J Clin Nutr* 1995; **62**:1239-44.

[292] Moynihan P, Adamson A, Rugg-Gunn A, Appleton D, Butler T. Dietary sources of calcium and the contribution of flour fortification to total calcium intake in the diets of Northumbrian adolescents. *Br J Nutr* 1996; **75**:495-505.

[293] Mills A, Tyler HA. *Food and nutrient intakes of British infants aged 6-12 months*. London: HMSO, 1992.

[294] Department of Health. *The Diets of British Schoolchildren*. Report on Health and Social Subjects: 36. London: HMSO, 1989.

[295] Bull N. Dietary habits of 15 - 25 year olds. *Hum Nutr: Appl Nutr* 1985; **39A**(suppl 1):1-68.

[296] Schofield C, Stewart J, Wheeler EF. The diets of pregnant and post-pregnant women in different social groups in London and Edinburgh: calcium, iron, retinol, ascorbic acid and folic acid. *Br J Nutr* 1989; **62**:363-77.

[297] Thompson B, Skipper D, Fraser C, Hewitt A, Hunter D. Dietary intake of Aberdeen primigravidae in 1950/51 and 1984/85. *J Hum Nutr Diet* 1989; **2**:345-59.

[298] Anderson AS, Campbell D, Shepherd R. Nutrition knowledge, attitude to healthier eating and dietary intake in pregnant compared to non-pregnant women. *J Hum Nutr Diet* 1993; **6**:335-53.

[299] Anderson AS, Campbell D, Shepherd R. The influence of dietary advice on nutrient intake during pregnancy. *Br J Nutr* 1995; **73**:163-77.

[300] Black AE, Wiles SJ, Paul AA. The nutrient intake of pregnant and lactating mothers of good socio-economic status in Cambridge. *Br J Nutr* 1986; **56**:59-72.

[301] Caughey P, Seamen C, Parry D, Farquhar D, MacLennan WJ. Nutrition of old people in sheltered housing. *J Hum Nutr Diet* 1994; **7**:263-8.

[302] Maisey S, Loughridge J, Southon S, Fulcher R. Variation in food group and nutrient intake with day of the week in an elderly population. *Br J Nutr* 1995; **73**:359-73.

[303] Bunker VW, Lawson MS, Stansfield MF, Clayton BE. The intake and excretion of calcium, magnesium and phosphorus in apparently healthy elderly people and those who are housebound. *J Clin Exp Gerontol* 1989; **11**:71-86.

[304] Vir SC, Love AHG. Nutritional status of institutionalised and non-institutionalised aged in Belfast, Northern Ireland. *Am J Clin Nutr* 1979; **32**:1934-47.

[305] Doyle W, Crawford MA, Wynn AHA, Wynn SW. The association between maternal diet and birth dimensions. *J Nutr Med* 1990; **1**:9-17.

[306] Haste FM, Brooke OG, Anderson HR, Bland JM. The effect of nutritional intake on outcome of pregnancy in smokers and non-smokers. *Br J Nutr* 1991; **65**(3):347-54.

[307] Rogers I, Emmett P. Diet during pregnancy in a population of pregnant women in South West England. *Eur J Clin Nutr* 1998; **52**:246-50.

[308] Abraham R, Campbell-Brown M, Haines AP, North WR, Hainsworth V, McFadyen IR. Diet during pregnancy in an Asian community in Britain - energy, protein, zinc, copper and calcium. *Hum Nutr: Appl Nutr* 1985; **39**:23-35.

[309] Abraham R, Brown MC, North WR, McFadyen IR. Diets of Asian pregnant women in Harrow; iron and vitamins. *Hum Nutr: Appl Nutr* 1987; **41**:164-73.

[310] Weaver CM, Plawecki KL. Dietary calcium: adequacy of a vegetarian diet. *Am J Clin Nutr* 1994; **59**(suppl): 1238S-41S.

[311] Draper A, Lewis J, Malhotra N, Wheeler EF. The energy and nutrient intakes of different types of vegetarian: a case for supplements? *Br J Nutr* 1993; **69**:3-19.

[312] Warrington S, Storey DM. Comparative studies on Asian and Caucasian children. 2. Nutrition, feeding practices and health. *Eur J Clin Nutr* 1988; **42**:69-80.

[313] Foster K, Lader D, Cheesbrough S. *Infant Feeding 1995*. London: The Stationery Office, 1997.

[314] Lawson M, Thomas M, Hardiman A. Iron status of Asian children aged two years living in England. *Arch Dis Child* 1998; **78**:420-426.

[315] Lawson M, Thomas M. Low vitamin D status of Asian two year olds living in England. *BMJ* 1998 (in press).

[316] Poskitt EME, Cole TJ, Lawson DEM. Diet, sunlight and 25-hydroxy vitamin D in healthy children and adults. *BMJ* 1979; **1**:221-3.

[317] Lester E, Skinner RK, Wills MR. Seasonal variation in serum 25-OH vitamin D in the elderly in Britain. *Lancet* 1977; **i**:979.

[318] Davies M, Mawer EB, Hann JT, Taylor JL. Seasonal changes in the biochemical indices of vitamin D deficiency in the elderly: a comparison of people in residential homes, long-stay wards and attending a day-hospital. *Age Ageing* 1986; **15**:77-83.

[319] Health Education Authority. *The Balance of Good Health*. London: Health Education Authority, 1996.

[320] Webb AR, Pilbeam C, Hanafin N, Holick MF. An evaluation of the relative contributions of exposure to sunlight and diet to the circulating concentrations of 25-hydroxyvitamin D in an elderly nursing home population in Boston. *Am J Clin Nutr* 1990; **51**:1075-81.

[321] Prentice AM, Jebb SA. Obesity in Britain: gluttony or sloth? *BMJ* 1995; **311**:437-9.

Table A1.1 Dietary Reference Values for calcium for populations groups in different countries (mg/d)

Population group	UK RNI[1]	EU PRI[2]	French ANC[3]	Nordic NR[4]	USA RDA[5]	Canadian RNI[6]	USA/Canadian AI[7]	Aust[8]/NZ RDI[9]
0-6 m	525	nvs	400	360	400	breastfed 250	210 formula fed 375	breast fed 300 formula fed 500
7-12 m	525	400	600	540	600	400 (5-12m)	270	550
1-3 y	350	400	600	600	800	500 (1y) 550 (2-3y)	500	700
4-6 y	450	400	700	600	800	600	800	800
7-10 y	550	550	700 (7-9y)	700	800	700 (7-9y)	800 (7-8y) 1300 (9-10y)	900F, 800M (8-11y)
11-14 y M	1000	1000	1000 (10-12y) 1200(13-14 y)	900	1200	900 (10-12y) 1100 (13-15y)	1300	1200 (12-15y)
11-14 y F	800	800	1000(10-12 y) 1200(13-14 y)	900	1200	1100 (10-12y) 1000 (13-15y)	1300	1000 (12-15y)
15-18 y M	1000	1000	1200	900	1200	900 (16-18y)	1300	1000 (16-18y)
15-18 y F	800	800	1200	900	1200	700 (16-18y)	1300	800 (16-18y)
19-50 y	700	700	900-1200	800-900	1200 (<24y) 800 (<25+y)	800M, 700F	1000	800
50+ y	700	700	1200	800	800	800	1200	1000F (54+y), 800M
Pregnancy	no extra	no extra	1200	900	1200	+500 (18y and below only)	+300 (18y and below only)	+300
Lactation	+550	1200	1200	1200	1200	+500 (18y and below only)	+300 (18y and below only)	+400

Notes: nvs = no value set
m = months
y = years
F = females / M = males
RNI (UK) = Reference Nutrient Intake
EU PRI = European Union Population Reference Intake

ANC = Apport Nutritionnel Conseillé
NR = Nutrition Recommendations
RDA = Recommended Dietary Allowance
RNI (Canada) = Recommended Nutrient Intake
AI = Adequate Intake
RDI = Recommended Dietary Intake

Table A1.2 Dietary Reference Values for vitamin D for populations groups in different countries (µg/d)

Population group		Country					
	UK RNI[1]	EU PRI[2]	French ANC[3]	Nordic NR[4]	USA RDA[5]	Canadian RNI[6]	USA/Canadian AI[7]
0-6 m	8.5	0-10	10	5	7.5	10***	5
7-12 m	7	0-10	10	5	10	10***	5
1-3 y	7	0-10	10	5	10	10 (1-2y) 5 (3y)	5
4-6 y	0*	0-10	10	5	10	5	5
7-10 y	0*	0-10	10 (7-9y)	5	10	2.5	5
11-14 y M	0*	0-10	10-15 (1-12y) 10 (13-14y)	5	10	2.5 (10-12y) 5 (13-14y)	5
11-14 y F	0*	0-10	10-15 (10-12y) 10 (13-14y)	5	10	5 (10-14y)	5
15-18 y M	0*	0-10	10	5	10	5	5
15-18 y F	0*	0-10	10	5	10	5 (15y) 2.5 (16-18y)	5
19-50y	0*	0-10	10	5	5-10	2.5	5
50+ y	10**	0-10	12	10	5	5	10 (51-70y) 15 (> 70y)
Pregnancy	10	0-10	20	10	10	2.5	5
Lactation	10	0-10	15	10	10	2.5	5

Notes:
* certain at-risk individuals may require dietary vitamin D
** for the population aged 65+ years only
*** An additional intake of 10µg/day is recommended for infants who are living in the far north of Canada during winter
m = months
y = years
F = females / M = males
RNI (UK) = Reference Nutrient Intake
EU PRI = European Union Population Reference Intake

ANC = Apport Nutritionnel Conseillé
NR = Nutrition Recommendations
RDA = Recommended Dietary Allowance
RNI (Canadian) = Reference Nutrient Intake
AI = Adequate Intake

Note:
New Zealand recommendations for vitamin D are not included as no reference value is set for dietary vitamin D. Australia recommend that those who are housebound could benefit from an oral intake of 10µg vitamin D/day if they are not exposed for 1-2 hours per week to direct sunlight in summer.

115

References

1.	Department of Health. *Dietary Reference Values for Food Energy and Nutrients for the United Kingdom.* Report on Health and Social Subjects: 41. London: HMSO, 1991.

2.	Commission of the European Communities. *Nutrient and energy intakes for the European Community.* Reports of the Scientific Committee for Food (31st series). Luxembourg: Office for Official Publications of the European Communities, 1993.

3.	Dupin H, Abraham J, Giachetti I. *Apports Nutritionnels Conseillés Pour la Population Française.* 2nd Edition. Paris: TEC and DOC Lavoisier, 1992.

4.	No. 1 Nordic Council of Ministers. Nordic Nutrition Recommendations 1996. *Scand J Nutr* 1996; **40**:161-165.

5.	National Research Council (U.S.). Subcommittee on the Tenth Edition of the RDAs. *Recommended dietary allowances.* Food and Nutrition Board, Commission on Life Sciences. National Research Council, 10th rev. ed. Washington, D.C.: National Academy of Life Sciences, 1989.

6.	Scientific Review Committee. Authority of the Minister of National Health and Welfare. *Nutrition Recommendations.* The Report of the Scientific Review Committee. Canada: Minister of Supply and Services, 1990.

7.	Institute of Nutrition Food and Nutrition Board. *Dietary Reference Intakes for Calcium, Phosphorus, Magnesium, Vitamin D, and Fluoride.* Washington: National Academy Press, 1997.

8.	National Health and Medical Research Council. *Recommended Dietary Intakes for use in Australia.* Canberra: Australian Government Publishing Service, 1991.

9.	Nutrition Taskforce (New Zealand). *Food for Health.* Report of the Nutrition Taskforce. Wellington: Department of Health, 1991.

Annex 2

Dietary Reference Values for Food Energy and Nutrients for the United Kingdom[1]

Paragraphs from the above report from COMA have been reproduced below to clarify the interpretation of Dietary Reference Values. See para 4.2.2 in this report.

1.3.11   For most nutrients the Panel found insufficient data to establish any of these DRVs with great confidence. There are inherent errors in some of the data, for instance in individuals' reports of their food intake, and the day-to-day variation in nutrient intakes also complicates interpretation. Even given complete accuracy of a dietary record, its relation to habitual intake remains uncertain, however long the recording period. The food composition tables normally used to determine nutrient intake from dietary records contain a number of assumptions and imperfections. Furthermore, there is uncertainty about the relevance of many biological markers, such as serum concentrations of a nutrient, as evidence of an individual's 'status' for that nutrient. Thus uncertainties relating to the appropriate parameter by which to assess the requirement, to the completeness of the database for any nutrient, and to the precision and accuracy of dietary intake data lead to the need to make judgements.

1.3.12   Equally, when nutrient intakes are measured there is demonstrable inter-individual variation, which is not necessarily related to the variation in requirements. Figure 1.2 demonstrates a distribution of intakes identical to the distribution of requirements but where any individual's intake is not necessarily the same as his own requirement. An individual whose intake is at point a - the LRNI - may be meeting his requirements for a nutrient, but it is highly probable that he is not. Similarly it is just possible, but very improbable, that an individual consuming a nutrient at point c - the RNI - will be consuming insufficient amounts of that nutrient. Whatever parameter is used the risk of deficiency in an individual at a given intake will vary from virtually zero at point c to virtually 100 per cent at point a. It should be recognised that the time course of the relationship between intake and status varies between different nutrients. For instance daily energy intakes should approximate requirements while assessment of intakes of some micronutrients needs to be integrated over days, weeks, or even longer. Furthermore not only may nutrients have effects on health at the time they are eaten, but there is growing evidence that diet may be one of the factors in early, even intrauterine, life which has an influence on later health in adult life.

1.3.13   If the distribution of intakes in a group of individuals is identical to that of their requirements for a nutrient it is probable that some with lower intakes will have higher requirements and vice versa. If there is no correlation between intakes and requirements in a group, then an average intake equal to the EAR carries a substantial risk of deficiency in the group represented by the upper dotted line depicting risk (Figure). In order to avoid this risk completely, the distribution of intakes of the group would have to be such that the lowest intakes exceeded the highest requirements. If, as is likely, there is some correlation between intakes and requirements, then the higher that correlation the lower the risk. In fact, there may be relationships between intake and requirements on the basis of body size, which in part determines energy requirements and therefore energy (and food) intakes. The degree to which this occurs is not known. The lower dotted line in Figure 1.2 represents the Panel's assessment of the actual risk of deficiency in a group, taking account of this. Furthermore, apparent requirements of individuals at prevailing intake levels may not represent basal requirements. If intake by an individual falls below the usual intake, there may be adaptive mechanisms which reduce the risk of deficiency but which may not be fully effective until a period of time has elapsed. This effect varies between different nutrients.

Reference

Department of Health. *Dietary Reference Values for Food Energy and Nutrients for the United Kingdom.* Report on Health and Social Subjects: 41. London: HMSO, 1991.

Figure Dietary intakes and risk of deficiency[1]

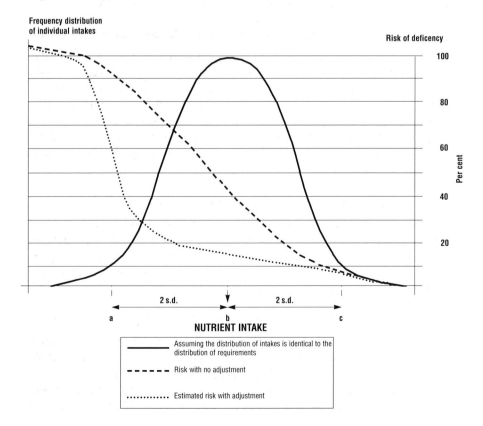

Annex 3

Monitoring dietary intakes and/or nutritional status in the UK

1. **National Food Survey (NFS)[1]**

This survey, commissioned by the Ministry of Agriculture, Fisheries and Food is an enquiry into the amounts and costs of food obtained by private households in Britain and of its nutrient content. The survey began in 1940 and since 1996 also covers Northern Ireland. About 8000 households, selected to be nationally representative, take part in this survey each year. The householder keeps a seven day record of the description, quantity and cost of all food entering the home for human consumption. Information on confectionery, alcoholic and soft drinks brought home and all food and drink purchased and eaten outside of the home has been collected since 1992. The NFS provides information on long term trends in national food consumption and nutrient intakes and variations in intake by groups of the population. It cannot, however, provide information about the food consumption and nutrient intake of individuals within a population.

2. **The Food and Nutrient Intakes of British Infants aged 6 - 12 months[2]**

This study was commissioned by MAFF to ascertain the food and nutrient intakes of older infants in Britain and to determine differences by region, socio-economic groups and presence of other children in the family. Dietary information was collected by means of a seven day record in which all food and drink items were specified by common household measures and recorded in a diary, followed by an interview with a parent. In total, 258 from the 6-9 month age group and 230 from the 9-12 month age group participated in the study. Fieldwork was in November 1986.

3. **Children aged 6 months to 4½ years in Britain - 1967/68[3]**

In 1967 the Department of Health and Social Security studied 1,321 infants and young children in Britain who were selected to be nationally representative. Demographic information about this group as well as 7 day weighed food intake record and anthropometric measurements were collected. Some of the children had medical and dental examinations.

4. **National Diet and Nutrition Survey: Children Aged 1½ to 4½ years[4]**

This survey, commissioned by the Department of Health and MAFF was carried out between July 1992 and June 1993. It provided detailed information about diet and nutritional status for preschool children living in private households in Britain. A nationally representative sample of 1859 children aged 1½-4½ years participated in the survey and only one child per household was selected. The survey collected information about socio-demographic circumstances of the child's household, medication and eating and drinking habits; a weighed dietary record of all food and drink consumed over four consecutive days (including Saturday and Sunday); a record of bowel movements for the same four days; physical measurements of the child (weight, standing height, supine length for children under two years, mid-upper arm and head circumferences). A sample of blood was taken for analysis. The survey also included an oral health examination.

5. Vitamin D status of Children aged 2 years in Asian Families Living in England[5]

The Department of Health commissioned a survey of the early feeding practices in Asian families in England. 2275 newborn Asian (Indian, Pakistani and Bangladeshi) infants born in autumn 1994 were included in the survey and compared with a group of 619 white infants born in the same localities. Information about how the babies were being fed was collected at age 6 weeks, 4, 9 and 15 months. At age 2 years the Asian children who could be traced, were asked to give a sample of blood for analysis of vitamin D and markers of iron status.

6. The Diets of British Schoolchildren[6]

This survey was undertaken between January and June 1983 to evaluate the dietary habits of older schoolchildren and the contribution made by school meals. Anthropometric measures (height and weight) and seven day weighed food records were collected. The data collected from 898 boys aged 10-11 years, 805 girls aged 10-11 years, 509 boys aged 14-15 years and 452 girls aged 14-15 years throughout Britain were analysed by age group, gender, region and socio-economic variables.

7. Survey of Dietary Habits of 15 to 25 year olds in Britain[7]

This study took place in March to June of 1982, and collected nationally representative data from 452 men and 461 women aged 15-25 years. Two week dietary diaries were used to record quantitative information (using household measures and standard portion size) about all food and drink consumed. Anthropometric (self-reported height and weight), lifestyle and socio-economic data were also collected.

8. Dietary and Nutritional Survey of British Adults[8]

This survey, commissioned jointly between the Department of Health and MAFF, collected dietary and nutritional status information on 2197 adults living in private households in Britain. It was carried out between October 1986 and August 1987. The participants, who were representative of the British population aged between 16 and 64 years (excluding pregnant women), kept a weighed food record of all food and drink consumed over seven consecutive days. Height, weight and blood pressure were determined and blood and urine (24 hour) samples were taken for analysis. Details of lifestyle characteristics (e.g. smoking, slimming, dietary supplement use) and socio-economic factors were also collected.

9. Nutrition and Health in Old Age[9]

This study, commissioned by the Department of Health and Social Security, in conjunction with the Scottish Home and Health Department, was first conducted in 1967/68 (on 879 subjects aged over 65 years), then much of the same sample population (379 subjects) were re-surveyed in 1972/73. Socio-economic, dietary (weighed seven day food and drink records), medical (to assess clinical signs of malnutrition), anthropometric (height, weight, upper arm circumference, and four skin fold measurements), biochemical and haematological (to assess sub-clinical signs of malnutrition from a range of nutrients, not including vitamin D) and radiological (x-ray of metacarpal bones for clinical assessment) information was obtained for each subject.

10. The National Diet and Nutrition Survey: people aged 65 years and over[10]

This survey, commissioned by the Department of Health and MAFF, was carried out between October 1994 and September 1995. It provided detailed information about the diet and nutritional status of 1687 people aged 65 years and older (1275 were free-living and 412 were living in institutions) in Britain. The participants were chosen to be nationally representative of Britain and kept a weighed record of all food and drink consumed over 4 consecutive days. This methodology was modified for the institutional group, and for a few free-living people who could not manage the weighing. Socio-economic, demographic and lifestyle characteristics were recorded. Anthropometric measurements of height, weight, mid-upper arm, waist and hip circumferences were taken as well as blood pressure, hand grip strength and a bowel movement record. Blood and urine samples were taken for analysis. The survey also included an oral health examination.

11. The National Diet and Nutrition Survey: young people aged 4-18 years

The fieldwork for this survey, commissioned by the Department of Health and MAFF, was conducted between January 1997 and January 1998. It will provide detailed information about the diet and nutritional status of young people aged 4-18 years in private households in Britain. The participants were chosen to be nationally representative of Britain and kept a record of all food and drink consumed over 7 consecutive days. Socio-economic, demographic and physical activity characteristics were recorded. Anthropometric measurements of height, weight, mid-upper arm circumference, waist and hip circumferences were taken as well as blood pressure and a bowel movement record. Blood and spot urine samples were taken for analysis. The survey also included an oral health examination. A report of the survey is expected to be published in 1999.

References

1.	Ministry of Agriculture, Fisheries and Food. *National Food Survey*. Annual reports of the National Food Survey Committee. London: HMSO/The Stationery Office, 1949-1997.

2.	Mills A, Tyler HA. *Food and nutrient intakes of British infants aged 6-12 months*. London: HMSO, 1992.

3.   Department of Health and Social Security. *A nutrition survey of preschool children, 1967-68.* Report on Health and Social Subjects: 10. London: HMSO, 1975.

4.   Gregory J, Collins DL, Davies PSW, Hughes JM, Clarke PC. *National Diet and Nutrition Survey: Children aged 1½ to 4½ years: Volume 1, Report of the diet and nutrition survey.* London: HMSO, 1995.

5.   Thomas M, Avery V. Infant Feeding in Asian Families. The Stationery Office, 1997.

6.   Department of Health. *The diets of British Schoolchildren.* Report on Health and Social Subjects: 36. London: HMSO, 1989.

7.   Bull   N. Dietary habits of 15-25 year olds. *Human Nutr Applied Nutr* 1985; **39A**(Suppl 1): 1-68.

8.   Gregory J, Foster K, Tyler HA, Wiseman M. *The dietary and nutritional survey of British adults.* London: HMSO, 1990.

9.   Department of Health and Social Security. *Nutrition and Health in Old Age.* Report on Health and Social Subjects: 19. London: HMSO, 1979.

10.   Finch S, Doyle W, Lowe C, Bates CJ, Prentice A, Smithers G, Clarke PC. *National Diet and Nutrition Survey: people aged 65 years and over. Volume 1: Report of the diet and nutrition survey.* London: The Stationery Office, 1998.

Annex 4

Table A4.1 The calcium content of some foods and dishes (mg)

Food	Description of average portion (where needed) and weight	Calcium content (mg) (approximate) Per portion	Calcium content (mg) (approximate) Per 100g
Whole milk	200g (1 glass)	230	115
Semi-skimmed/skimmed milk	200g (1 glass)	240	120
Cheddar cheese	40g (medium chunk)	290	720
Cottage cheese	112g (plain, small pot	80	75
Low fat, fruit yoghurt	125g (1 pot)	190	150
White bread*	36g (1 slice)	40	110
Brown bread*	36g (1 slice)	35	100
Wholemeal bread	36g (1 slice)	20	55
Baked beans	135g	70	55
Broccoli, boiled	85g	35	40
Cabbage, boiled	95g	30	35
1 egg, boiled	50g	30	55
Branflakes	30g (1 portion)	15	50
Composite dishes			
Rice pudding, canned	200g	190	
Cheese and tomato pizza*, medium	200g	360	
Cauliflower cheese	200g	240	
Cheesecake	120g	80	
Sardines in tomato sauce on toast*	50g sardines & 1 slice of white bread	255	
Cornflakes			
- with whole milk	30g cereal	120	
- with semi-skimmed/skimmed milk	& 100g milk	125	
1 cheddar cheese sandwich			
- with white bread*	14g soft margarine,	405	
- with wholemeal bread	45g cheese & 2 slices of bread	365	
1 cottage cheese sandwich			
- with white bread*	14g soft margarine,	115	
- with wholemeal bread	50g cottage cheese & 2 slices of bread	75	

*Fortified with calcium

123

Table A4.2 The vitamin D content of some foods and dishes (μg)

Food	Description of average portion (where needed) and weight	Vitamin D content (μg) (approximate) Per portion	Per 100g
Smoked mackerel	150g (1 medium)	12.0	8.0
Salmon, canned in brine	45g	7.7	17.0
Sardines, canned in tomato sauce	50g	4.0	8.0
Tuna, canned in brine	45g	1.8	4.0
1 egg, boiled	50g	0.9	1.7
Roast beef, lean topside	90g (1 slice)	0.7	0.8
Roast pork, lean loin	90g (1 slice)	0.7	0.8
Roast chicken	100g (1 slice)	0.2	0.2
Lambs liver, fried	100g	0.5	0.5
Butter, spread on 1 slice of bread	10g	0.08	0.8
Low fat spread* on 1 slice of bread	7g	0.6	8.4
Margarine*, soft on 1 slice of bread	7g	0.5	7.8
Cheddar cheese	40g (medium chunk)	0.1	0.3
Branflakes*	30g (1 portion)	0.6	2.1
Composite dishes			
Sardines in tomato sauce on toast*	50g sardines and	4.0	
- with soft margarine* 7g on toast	1 slice of bread	4.5	
Tuna mayonnaise sandwich	14g soft margarine,		
- with tuna in brine	45g tuna,	3.0	
- with tuna in oil	33g mayonnaise & 2 slices of bread	3.8	
Fortified breakfast cereal	30g cereal		
e.g. Rice Krispies*	100g milk		
- with whole milk		0.7	
- with semi-skimmed/skimmed milk		0.6	

*Fortified with vitamin D